Modern Asian Mom
A memoir about fertility, motherhood, and life

Dr. Juliet Dang

Modern Asian Mom

Second Edition

ISBN: 978-1-965142-64-6 (Paperback)
ISBN: 978-1-965142-65-3 (Hardback)
Library of Congress Control Number: 2025918790

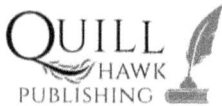

QUILL HAWK PUBLISHING

Edmond, OK

Dedicated to my mother, Anna.
Thank you for everything.

Table of Contents

Preface

Although this book is titled Modern Asian Mom (MAM), the experiences many women go through are universal. Some other cultures and races share similar traditions, practices, superstitions, events, traumas, dramas, etc.

My fertility journey is not exclusive; some women can empathize with these events. Some women have gone through several versions of hell trying to conceive and have never come out victorious. My heart goes to all the women who feel like they have failed because their reproductive organs did not live up to personal and societal expectations. We are all people and not just mere vessels for procreation. What WE think, feel, want, and do matters more than anything—much more important than continuing our legacy.

My biggest thanks go to my husband, Micah. I can "do it all" because he is a true partner and a terrific father. I am lucky that I found the second love of my life who helped me to have the third love of my life. Specifically, I am the first love of my life, which shall always be. Loving oneself is imperative to having a healthy and balanced dynamic with anyone in our lives (cliché yet true).

My book, which began as a fertility memoir, naturally evolved into other aspects of my life. I also felt naturally inclined to include the experiences and stories of other mothers. Hopefully, my collective experiences and those of other mothers will provide readers with helpful insights and reminders that they are not alone. We don't realize that the tiny bubbles we reside in are connected with invisible silk to each other. The pulls, tightens, and releases are felt in the interconnected web of womanhood, resulting in a universal sisterhood. One of the most important learnings of my journey is that gestures of support and empathy in any predicament are crucial for resolution.

1. The Modern Asian Mom

I watched the third season of Bling Empire LA, and Kelly spoke about her surface-level relationship with her mother and how she would love to have a meaningful connection with her. She mentioned feeling that while growing up, nothing was ever good enough, and there was so much pressure to be the best at everything, i.e., school, ballet, piano, etc. Perhaps the most crucial aspect she shared was that they never spoke about their feelings.

Many of us who grew up in Asian households can empathize with this sentiment, and as we become adults, it becomes clearer why our parents do not speak to us like we are their confidantes or friends. Our parents don't fall far from the very tree they came from, plus our grandparents were most likely not open books nor ones to wear their hearts on their sleeves. The older generations grew up in a different atmosphere—a seemingly colder culture, more non-communicative and non-empathetic. Not only do we need to consider the trauma they may have endured, but many were first-generation immigrants, leaving war-torn nations to start over in a new country.

Kelly and Kane from *Bling Empire LA* spoke about how hard it was to tell their parents they loved them because it was never a practice in their homes. It's funny how I can relate to this, but oppositely—my mother always told me she loved me, but for some reason, I found it difficult to say it back. Perhaps my inability to say "I love you" came from other places, such as resentment for my mother's strictness or her constant helicoptering. Maybe I wanted to save the moment for my lame high school boyfriends. I felt embarrassed to say those three words, and it still evades me as to why.

It was touching to watch Kelly and her mother break through the surface layers to speak on a deeper level and share their vulnerabilities. Just thinking about it made me feel awkward and uncomfortable because

I, too, had a very shallow relationship with my mother. I truly wish that my mother were alive today so that we could work on our communication and become closer. Just writing about this makes me squirm around uncomfortably.

Our relationship with our mothers can shape how we become mothers to our children, whether we like it or not. We have innate reflexes to react to behaviors we don't accept, though what is more difficult is the intentional act of compassion and empathy with the addition of boundaries. The term "boundary" is non-existent in Asian families; the same silk scarf that holds the family together can also strangle. Although we Asians may seem to be quite resilient, there is always a breaking point.

So, what exactly is a Modern Asian Mom (MAM)? I don't believe there is a straightforward answer to this; however, at the end of my memoir, I attempt to define it to the best of my ability. Throughout this book, we delve into various situations, primarily my own personal experiences, as well as those I have heard about, where I notice certain trends emerging or topics that I think are worth discussing. It is interesting to see how other mothers react to a variety of events. The trials and tribulations are perhaps not primarily different, but perhaps we now react more modernly (or some of us try to). Though, it's hard for the apple not to fall far from the tree. Our mother's voice is the first thing we hear from within the womb, constantly reverberating.

Growing up in an Asian household is a unique experience that should not be taken lightly. Through countless conversations with friends and observing the dynamics of different households, growing up Asian can be pretty dysfunctional. The intergenerational trauma, language barriers, cultural differences, conditional love, high expectations, high standards, and high pressure—all of it makes you, and then eventually breaks you. The experiences we grow up with shape us and entirely affect how we react, behave, and, most importantly, sculpt our self-worth. Hence, who we end up with and how much we put up with is directly connected to our upbringing.

For example, there are still expectations in today's modern times for Asian women to be dutiful, obedient, loyal wives and daughters-in-law. These engrained old-school practices from the first-generation immigrants die hard. What we want doesn't matter; this is a recipe for disaster because when we dare to stand up for ourselves, this is met with gaslighting and guilt-tripping.

Social media is a trove of advice, information sharing, gossip, drama, all of it! It's entertaining, eye-opening, shocking, yet there are even frightful stories of what some mothers go through. There are also a lot of trolls. The lack of compassion from some people is extremely disappointing to witness. What was also surprising was realizing that common sense for one person wasn't the same for the next.

With age comes greater wisdom, hopefully, and I have learned that people's struggles and realities are circumstances we may not be fully able to comprehend. Support can mean the world to someone, even in the form of affirmation.

2. To Be a Parent

"Make sure your children's academic, emotional, psychological, mental, spiritual, physical, nutritional, and social needs are met while being careful not to overstimulate, underestimate, improperly medicate, helicopter, or neglect them in a screen-free, processed foods-free, plastic-free, body-positive, socially conscious, egalitarian but also authoritative, nurturing but fostering of independence, gentle but not overly permissive, pesticide-free, two-story, multilingual home preferable in a cul-de-sac with a backyard. And don't forget the coconut oil."
— Dr. Siggie Cohen, Child Development Specialist

Women can do it all and have it all. Right?

So, you know how you have a concrete plan for your life and every intention to execute that plan with no obstacles? The warning that I had to "have kids by age thirty-five or else" rang in my ears like a constant fire alarm. Like, if it didn't happen by thirty-five, I was at risk of never having children—ever. Thus, I was adamant that by thirty-five, I should be pregnant to avoid the risk of my ovaries becoming entirely "geriatric." The whole notion of your womb turning into cobwebs before you are even ready to have children is an Instant Pot; it's like a nagging pressure being built up that instills fear, anxiety, and guilt. You could blow up in a bad way (outcome = no baby) or a good way (outcome = baby).

In the Spring of 2015, I was writing my PhD dissertation and was scheduled to defend it in June. I was about to turn thirty-four and realized that becoming accidentally pregnant wouldn't be that bad. Thus, after a decade of popping birth control pills, I stopped. I spent twelve years in regular school and another twelve years in university. It was time to start a new chapter of my life. The time and energy I invested in my education were akin to climbing a few mountains. I loved being a

4

student, but it was time to shift to other projects. Perhaps I was somewhat past the point of being horrified of having an *alien-like leech* grow inside me.

After graduating with a PhD in Oral Biology, it took me six months to land a job, which was in Pharma marketing. The CEO was insane, and I was fired within five months. Lemons turned into lemonade as I could go to Switzerland without commotion and receive a World Research Award for my work on human papillomaviruses in head and neck cancers. Sunstar Butler, the company that sponsored the awards and ceremony, spared no expense. It was quite the procession with a traditional Swiss cowbell choreography (an interesting traditional dance where men wave giant cowbells in front of their crotch) and flag-throwing Swiss ladies, all taking place inside Basel Stadium, where football (soccer) matches occur. It was a spectacle; I felt like a queen receiving my crown.

Fast forward to the Fall of 2016, when I finally had the patience and nerve to purchase an ovulation test kit while still on a manic job hunt. I had no idea how to decipher whether I was ovulating, what the signs were, or the actual biology of it all, and I was a bloody scientist! I didn't need to know all the technical details because I thought getting pregnant would be simple. How hard could it be to get pregnant, right? Since I wasn't working, my husband Micah and I visited Italy and Malta. I thought for sure I would get pregnant going to such romantic destinations.

I read the directions and dutifully collected my urine sample every morning beginning on day eight or so of my cycle. By the way, learning to keep track of your cycle is paramount. Day one is the first day of your period, and ovulation is typically days twelve to fourteen. However, I have heard it could be earlier. At that point, I didn't know the signs I should be looking for in terms of consistency of vaginal discharge during ovulation. Unfortunately, I didn't realize until three years later that monitoring your discharge is a more accurate indicator than ovulation test kits.

According to my tests, I was ovulating around day twelve. A European vacation didn't seem to do the trick, and I believed that all it took was taking these tests to become pregnant. I mean, how difficult can this be?

Wasn't this what my body was made for? Having babies when the time was right? When I was actually ready for it? Pah!

After a few testing cycles, I stopped and became tired of the routine. If it happens, it happens—the words of affirmation you tell yourself to trick your mind and body into thinking you were so nonchalant about it when, of course, all you could think about is, why haven't I gotten pregnant yet? Was there something wrong with me? I had no clue, but we headed to Japan for the Sakura Festival in the Spring of 2017 since I was not pregnant.

By June of 2017, I had landed my dream career as a medical science liaison. It took me a year to obtain it. At last, we could be real *DINKs* (dual income, no kids)! My "American dreams" were coming to fruition, eh? The Canadian in me was laughing as I had once said, "I will never live in the States."

3. Dr. Doogie

By Fall 2017, I had decided to get an OBGYN and sought other options. Coincidentally, I was scheduled with the same OBGYN as one of my close girlfriends, who had the same birthday. Throughout our friendship, we discovered quirky similarities and coincidences, e.g., our dogs have the same birthday, my husband and her sister have the same birthday, we own the same Club Monaco skirt from fifteen years ago, and so on.

Dr. Doogie seemed relatively young (hence the alias referencing the main character in the ABC sitcom *Doogie Howser, M.D.*, an American medical sitcom that ran from 1989 to 1993), perhaps similar in age to myself, and after we told her our history the first thing she blurted out was, "Just do IVF, and you will be guaranteed to have a healthy baby!"

I sat in shock because I was there to seek other options before going full-on with In Vitro Fertilization. I felt IVF should be my last option, right? I sat there and stared blankly for a bit while Micah asked Dr. Doogie about testing his sperm and turkey basting, aka intrauterine insemination (IUI). This process involves the collection of sperm, washing it with reagents, spinning it down so that it is super concentrated, and then injecting it into your cervix when they think you are ovulating. We left Dr. Doogie's office in a daze with a series of scheduled blood tests and a sperm analysis.

During our follow-up appointment, Dr. Doogie indicated that everything looked pretty normal, except the morphology of Micah's sperm looked a bit weird. Her "young," naïve, and slightly inconsiderate tone sent my honey into an internal fury. She continued to explain that sometimes sperm look weird, but that doesn't mean they cannot complete their duty. After that appointment, Micah did not want to see Dr. Doogie again.

I think most men are pretty sensitive when it comes to the quality and function of their reproductive parts. I would take offense, too, if I were told my eggs looked ugly. But then again, what's the difference when my eggs are deemed geriatric by age thirty-five?

Since everything on paper seemed pretty okay, we proceeded to keep trying, but in a more relaxed manner. I didn't routinely keep track of my ovulation, didn't take prenatal pills, and never really thought about what it meant to get my body in a pre-pregnancy state. We planned a trip to Norway and the French Riviera for the summer of 2018, saying again that this was our last big trip before we sought other fertility assistance options.

in·fer·til·i·ty
/ ˌinfərˈtilədē/
inability to conceive children or young.

I have a big problem with utilizing the term "infertility" for women who have fully functioning reproductive organs with perfectly normal hormonal levels and who, for unknown reasons, have not become pregnant yet. Just because you haven't been pregnant doesn't mean you don't have viable eggs. I feel the traditional definition is too general, and there are varying levels of inability to conceive. There seems to be a spectrum. Perhaps the fallopian tubes are blocked by mucus, restricting sperm from traveling to the "golden egg." This is a physical blockage, not a woman who should be labeled as infertile. For women who have to go through IVF and use their eggs, I would not consider them to be infertile. This definition is archaic and does not fully encompass the complexity of the female reproductive system nor the nuances of procreation.

According to the World Health Organization (WHO), Infertility is "a *disease* of the reproductive system defined by the failure to achieve a clinical pregnancy after twelve months or more of regular unprotected sexual intercourse." (Reference: WHO-ICMART glossary) So, WHO thinks I have a disease because I haven't become pregnant in a bloody year? Not only was I considered geriatric in my reproductive years, but now I had a disease. How much worse can we feel as women who are trying to conceive? These clinical definitions are incomprehensible. I know plenty of women who hadn't conceived until their forties. Did that mean they were then cured of their so-called "disease?" I couldn't help but wonder if male OBGYNs defined this term.

Did you know J. Marion Sims, a white man who did experimental surgery on enslaved Black women without anesthesia, founded gynecology? There are no words to describe this horror, and I am so glad that NYC took down his statue in 2018. If more women healthcare professionals were part of actually doing gynecological research, I believe we would have more answers and more knowledge on women's reproductive health. The same goes for men's reproductive health. How many studies are being done on this population? It is convenient to blame the woman and her eggs because we don't have the data to clarify further.

4. When Are You Guys Having Kids?

Before I turned thirty-five, I was okay with answering this question because I felt no pressure during this time. I was in graduate studies for seven years and then had to obtain a job, so I was still working on myself and my dream career. The answer was always the same: "Ya, I have to get a job first, and then we can have kids," or "Ya, we aren't preventing, so you never know what will happen."

Once I turned thirty-five, the pressure was on because I hadn't become pregnant yet. People around me said, "You need to have kids now," like it was as easy as going to the kitchen and making a bloody sandwich. This sort of commentary from males was even more infuriating because they were entirely ignorant of the fact that conceiving was not an easy and immediate task.

According to a 2004 study by Henri Leridon, PhD, an epidemiologist with the French Institute of Health and Medical Research, of women trying to get pregnant without using fertility drugs or IVF (source – Wikipedia):

At age 30, 75% will have a conception ending in a live birth within one year, and 91% will have a conception ending in a live birth within four years.

At age 35, 66% will have a conception ending in a live birth within one year, and 84% will have a conception ending in a live birth within four years.

At age 40, 44% will have a conception ending in a live birth within one year, and 64% will have a conception ending in a live birth within four years.

This study utilized a computer simulation model of reproduction to estimate the probabilities. Thus, it had its limitations. Truly, modern, real-world studies completed on women, men, and fertility seem to be quite limited still. In general, the studies I scanned seemed to indicate that women in their mid-30s have more difficulties conceiving naturally compared to younger women and have a higher risk of miscarriage and birth abnormalities.

Turkey Basting

We came back to Dr. Doogie after our Europe trip in the Summer of 2018 and scheduled an IUI (intrauterine insemination, aka turkey basting). I wasn't prescribed Letrozole the first time, which is technically a treatment for breast cancer but used off-label for fertility assistance purposes. The drug suppresses estrogen production to trigger the pituitary gland to produce hormones for ovary stimulation. Thus, the hope was to produce more than one or higher quality follicle to release the ever-so-coveted "golden" eggs.

I came in for an ultrasound on day twelve of my cycle, where the nurse placed what looked like an enormous dildo in my vagina. Thank god only the tip was inserted right at the opening. The screen showcased circular shapes, and it appeared that I produced approximately three follicles per ovary. The nurse thought I needed to return for another ultrasound as she wanted my follicles and uterine lining to mature more. We came back the next day, and my left ovary seemed larger, with more mature follicles about sixteen to nineteen millimeters in diameter. The uterine lining thickened slightly; thus, the nurse okayed the IUI for the next day.

In the morning, Micah produced a sperm sample. The lab spun down his sample and washed it with some reagents to filter out the non-alpha and "weird-looking" sperm. We returned in a couple of hours, and I was now legs up in the stirrups. A nurse showed me the little needle that would be inserted into my cervix with the spun-down sperm concentrate that would be injected up into my fallopian tubes to hopefully meet a perfectly formed, viable, high-quality egg. The procedure was not super uncomfortable; it was just a twinge of cramping, and then it was done. I laid there with Micah by my side for fifteen whole minutes.

Well, I guess this is it, I thought. *My freedom will no longer be mine. I will be a slave to the parasitic leech inside of me.* I was thirty-seven, so it was already two years past the deadline I had set for myself. Truly, I should have been on child number two by then. I hadn't become pregnant yet, but the IUI would undoubtedly do the trick. I just knew it!

Two weeks went by, and I started my period like clockwork.

I remember two distinct conversations I had with two friends on separate occasions. Friend #1, Kate, and I were chatting about our mutual friend who hadn't been able to conceive for quite some time. The conversation went something like this:

Kate: We can't always have what we want in life. Like, she has a lovely house and chickens! Where are my chickens? I can't have everything I want either.

Me: But you are pregnant. Having chickens and being able to have babies are not the same thing.

Kate: Well, sometimes life is unfair.

I don't know if it was the pregnancy hormones, but this lady's thinking was wack! Chickens and babies are not equal.

Friend #2, Fiona, and I discussed how hard it was to conceive.

Fiona: I feel sorry for you and Stephanie.

Me: What? Why?

Fiona: Because you guys aren't pregnant yet, and there's a lot of pressure.

Me: It's tough, but I don't need you to feel sorry for me.

Now I had a pity party, how wonderful. The last thing I needed was for someone to feel sorry or pity me. It made me feel worse about myself that these were the thoughts surrounding a woman's inability to conceive. Of course, Fiona only had the best intentions, but this added to another level of feeling helpless.

5. Human Pin Cushion

I was told acupuncture could assist significantly in conceiving. So, I thought I would give it a go since I would be doing more IUIs in the future. During my first appointment, Lauryl asked me a series of health questions regarding my diet, exercise routine, hours of sleep, stress levels, etc. Her advice was:

It would be best if you didn't skip breakfast. A tea latté is not nutritious enough. No more cold salads, as you want to create heat in your tummy area; thus, cooked vegetables are better. You need to eat a little more meat, and you don't have to eat a lot, just more. Your lifestyle generally seems busy with your day job and all the side gigs (i.e., art, modeling, acting, and community activities). It would help if you were taking it easy, reading more books, or taking more naps. The color of your blood during your menstrual cycle indicates some stagnancy. (I was under the impression that crimson was a brilliant period color.) We want the blood to be a bright red with little to no clots. Acupuncture will help to bring more blood flow to the proper areas and reset your chi.

What Lauryl advised translated into her wanting me to turn into a boring, chubby, internally non-stagnant, plain Jane. The acupuncture itself was interesting. There are some places in the body where the pin creates a dull, throbbing sensation, which means my chi needs to be reset at that spot. Each appointment was not always the same. I had pins placed on my feet, legs, tummy (right before ovulation), arms, hands, ear canal, neck, forehead, and the top of my head. I usually fell asleep, and whenever I jerked any muscles, it would hurt where the pin was. Thus, I had to be extra careful with any sudden movements. For the most part, I was stuck for almost an hour trying to relax.

Time to Get Serious

By the Autumn of 2018, I was dead serious about getting pregnant. I went to see Lauryl almost every week or at least every two weeks. I modified my diet according to her suggestions, tried to back off on my side projects as much as possible, and watched more TV to "relax." I had another IUI scheduled for October and even had a new nurse practitioner who was this cute young red-headed woman with a nervous giggle. I had to get a hysterosalpingography (HSG) test completed, where they shot a fluorescent dye up my cervix to see if any of my fallopian tubes were blocked. This procedure might help to clear up any mucus blockages as well. Some pain occurred when they shot the dye up, but it subsided in a minute. (The tech asked me if I was okay because I didn't make a peep when they injected me; they thought my lack of response was regal.) The X-ray machine presented a picture of my tubes, and they all looked clear. The procedure was completed in less than ten minutes. I was given a pad at the end because the orange dye would leak for twenty-four hours. *PSA: If you have sex that same day, you will stain the sheets orange; thus, it is not a good idea.*

My IUI was scheduled a few days after the HSG. This time I was put on Letrozole to help my follicles grow bigger. I took these pills for five days starting on day three of my period. At the ultrasound appointment, Kelsey, the giggly redhead, measured about three mature follicles per ovary. The following day, Micah produced a robust sample, and a few hours later, I came in to have the spun-down concentrate injected into my cervix once again. I was so excited because I knew my tubes would be clear of mucus from the HSG! This time, it was bound to work! I again lay for fifteen minutes on the table after the IUI, both of us fiddling on our phones. I gave it an extra five minutes of wait time to be sure. Two weeks later, the crimson wave came into town, but I was not giving up! So, I scheduled another IUI in November.

I continued diligently making acupuncture appointments and increased my protein intake with cooked veggies. I was binge-watching on Netflix like no other now! *Soon, I will be a big, lazy sack of potatoes with the happiest follicles.* It was fascinating because I essentially halted my extra projects and endeavors only to pick up another one that would create more work once done, incubating and launching out into the world.

My November IUI wasn't successful yet again. After this round, I decided to wait a bit and not pressure myself too much. I scheduled another one in March of 2019 with no luck. At that point, I was nervous that maybe something was truly wrong with me. So, we took a break from the IUIs, and I concentrated solely on making my body as fertile as possible. We scheduled an appointment with PNW (Pacific Northwest) Fertility Clinic that summer to figure out a plan. If I had Micah on my medical insurance plan, we would most likely be covered for one round of IVF entirely. Thus, we opted to start IVF in December so I could have my egg retrieval in January when Micah would be officially switched over to my plan. This was my thought, and I would be damned if it didn't go accordingly.

We planned a trip to Europe that autumn as it would most likely be our last international vacation (for real now!). The plan was to head to Paris, Venice, quaint towns in the Dolomite regions, Salzburg, and Vienna. We have been on many trips before, but this was one of my favorites. There was magic in all of the places we visited. I had the chance to relax from our fertility project and eat nommy European cheeses to become more chubby. Our trip to Paris was too short, and we only had a day to see the Louvre, Tour d'Eiffel, and Champs-Élysées. Venice was such a sweet town and was picturesque. Once in Northern Italy, we stayed at a charming hotel spa that provided a half-board, where breakfast and dinner were provided. The meals were delectable.

All ingredients were local, and the options were grand. Europeans know how to have a proper relaxing vacation; Americans could learn something from them about self-care. The Dolomites are an epic mountain range originally part of the Austro-Hungarian Empire until the US stole it and gave it to Italy in 1918. Thus, the languages spoken in this region were multiple. Salzburg was the birthplace of Mozart, and I fell in love with its musical aura, which floated through the air. Vienna was a great city to shop in! With such a relaxing and fun vacay, my next round of eggs was bound to be extra viable and happy.

6. The Fertility Regimen

Since beginning acupuncture, I have added other lifestyle changes. My list of fertility action items included:

- Acupuncture weekly or bi-weekly
- Eat more meat
- Take a cocktail of supplements - fish oil, berberine, coQ10, vitamin D, vitamin C, probiotics, prenatal medicine
- Castor oil packs on my abdomen - putting a cloth saturated with castor oil on my tummy and putting a heat pack on top for an hour after my period up until ovulation
- Eat a cup of chi soup once daily, which helps reset the chi. Both you and your partner can do this. Here's the recipe and instructions:
  - Kombu
  - Wakame
  - Napa Cabbage
  - Leek
  - Mushrooms
  - Carrots
  - Kale
  - Lotus Root
  - Burdock root
  - Three-year aged miso

Take half of the miso and mix it with cold water. In a pot, from bottom to top, layer these ingredients, starting with the kombu and finishing with the miso on top of all the stacked ingredients. Add water about halfway and steam all the veggies until they are soft, then add more water to cover the veggies and boil for a bit more. I recommend making an extra-large pot, then aliquoting it and freezing several containers. You can add other veggies that are in season.

- Try not to fill my calendar with extraneous activities and take it easy
- Stay away from negative or toxic individuals, and make sure my circle of girlfriends consists of supportive and loving people
- Consume pineapple for an increase in uterine lining growth
- Consume durian when possible, as I read somewhere that it was the king of fruits and could help with fertility

Should Be Coming Anytime Now.

It was the week of Thanksgiving, and I was expecting my period to come soon. We drove to the Tricities in Eastern Washington, where Micah's dad lived, to spend quality time with the supernumerary Cain family. I prepared myself for the crimson wave and even felt cramping, so I thought it would soon start. We spent time with the family for a couple of days, which was a regular affair, and when we arrived back home in Seattle, I still hadn't gotten my period. I was usually never late, but I thought it would come at some point. *I can't be pregnant, though, right?* I had never been pregnant before, so why would I be now? I purchased a pregnancy test and was flabbergasted. It was positive for the first time in my life EVER. I showed Micah, and he was ecstatic! We wondered if our vacay time had a part to play since I was more relaxed. In general, I believed it was everything I did for the last year: acupuncture, diet change, chi soup, castor oil packs, and gaining some weight. I gained about ten pounds within a year. I also switched acupuncturists at the end of summer because Lauryl was going on maternity leave.

My new acupuncturist, Tate, was great! She had cool arm tattoos and was akin to a little witch pixie who could cure me of anything! Her recommendations were more extensive than Lauryl's and included action items for Micah. The ones that stood out were castor oil packs to stimulate blood circulation in the abdomen (which may boost a response in the ovaries), eating pineapple to produce a robust uterine lining, and eating soups to keep the body warm. Independent of this, I ate fresh durian. Most folks cannot appreciate this fruit because of its potent odor, but the taste of the fresh fruit is super nommy. It has a savory flair to me, and maybe that's why I enjoy it so much: I prefer umami items. It is easy to crack open the spiky things. Just Google it.

My weight gain was not due to just the diet but also the hormones I used for the IUI procedures. Truly, it was most likely a mixture of events and lifestyle modifications that led to my first natural pregnancy.

Becoming pregnant naturally felt like an accomplishment, and I never thought it would occur after all that time through my journey. It provided more faith that I could potentially have a successful pregnancy. I wanted to tell the world, but was reluctant in case something terrible occurred.

<u>What is Happening?</u>

Six weeks into my pregnancy, I began cramping and then saw some blood spotting, which went from pink to brown. I knew some spotting was expected, so I tried not to freak out.

Later on that week, Micah wanted to have sex, and I was up for it. However, it needed to be snappy because I had to fly out in a couple of hours. We both took our before-sex showers so I could decrease my risk of a UTI and hopped into bed. Amid our lovemaking, I noticed a blood stain on our sheets. We immediately stopped, and I saw some fresh blood. Of course, I freaked out a bit. The bleeding didn't continue after sex, and Micah thought I should call Dr. Doogie's office. I found an extra pregnancy test in my cabinet and decided to test myself just in case. I had only done two pregnancy tests, and that was on the very first day we found out, where I repeated the test for verification, like a true scientist would. I should have completed a triplicate - replication is essential in the lab.

I called Dr. Doogie's office to ask the nurse a question and described what had occurred. They took down some notes and said a nurse would call me back. I then needed to go to the washroom, so I took the pregnancy test and thanked the lord, baby Jesus Christ, and Mary Magdalene because it came out positive straight away. What I didn't know at the time was that your pregnancy hormones take a while to leave your body. Thus, a pregnancy test verifies you have pregnant hormones in your body, but a live fetus will only be confirmed via ultrasound.

I received a call from the nurse within thirty minutes. She had a series of questions for me:

Nurse: Did you see blood after having sex?

Me: No, during.

Nurse: When did you have intercourse?

Me: Today.

Nurse: What time?

Me: Around 3 pm.

Nurse: Where did you see the blood?

Me: I saw some on my partner and then on the bed sheets.

Nurse: Was the size on the sheets the size of a pea, a quarter, a baseball?

Me: More than a quarter.

Nurse: So, like a silver dollar?

Me: Ya around there. (I had no clue about the dimensions of a silver dollar.)

Nurse: Did the bleeding stop or continue?

Me: It stopped after we stopped having sex.

Nurse: Do you have any cramping?

Me: I feel a slight dull cramping, but feel fine in general.

Nurse: Your cervix tissue may be extra sensitive right now, which may be why the bleeding occurred. Generally, everything seems okay, but if you experience more bleeding, call us.

Me: I have to catch a flight tonight to Boise. Is it safe for me to do so?

Nurse: Let me ask Dr. Doogie. Hold for a few minutes, please.

Nurse: The doctor said you should be fine if you have stopped bleeding, and Boise does have emergency hospitals, so if you start bleeding, you need to go to one. Also, let us know if you think you should come in earlier than your appointment next week.

Me: Well, what do you think? Should I come in earlier? I would go based on your advice.

Nurse: Actually, I think you will be okay.

Me: Okay, thank you for all of the help.

Nurse: You're welcome. Take care.

Tate, my cute new acupuncturist, told me to be a potato until twelve weeks. My risk for miscarriage at my age caused me anxiety since I had never been pregnant before. I took every precaution in the bloody (no pun intended) book. Micah told me I could always reschedule my meeting and switch to a phone conference. I decided to play it safe. Plus, I felt exhausted and did not have the energy to walk up the stairs properly. There was no way I could walk efficiently through the airport terminals. Pregnant women are already put in a high-risk category, and at my "geriatric" reproductive age, I was like triple high-risk. I felt hungry and asked Micah to get me a truffle hamburger and fries.

Later, around midnight, I bled some more, about a couple of teaspoons' worth. I was more nervous and thought I was miscarrying. I woke up at 4:15 am, and the same two teaspoons of red blood appeared. There was no cramping, only a slight dull pain. I had my conference call at 7 am, which I rescheduled since I didn't fly into Boise. I felt exhausted and needed to rest quite often. More bleeding occurred after the call with a blob-clot-looking thing, and I apologized to what I thought was my miscarried baby. I called the nurse at my OBGYN's office. She said the blob/clot thing was most likely coagulated blood from the day before. Since I wasn't cramping and my bleeding was every few hours, we both decided it was okay to wait until my first appointment, which was in a week. The most they could do was run a blood test to check my HCG levels, but that would need to be repeated in forty-eight hours, and they were closed on Sunday. With the Christmas holidays, it wouldn't have worked. I thanked her and then got back to work on my computer.

During midday, the cramping got stronger and a bit more painful. The bleeding continued every few hours. I barely made it to my acupuncture appointment as I felt uncomfortable and weak. Tate was appalled that my OBGYN said it was okay for me to fly out the night before and said I made the right choice not to go. She listened to my recollection of the last twenty-four hours and said that it could go either way, meaning I may or may not be miscarrying, and most of the time, women who have these episodes go on to have their child.

There is an occurrence called "missed miscarriage," where the mother-to-be doesn't even know she is having one, and then on the other end of the spectrum, you have terrible cramps, and it all flushes out in one go. I was nestled in the unknown, where we didn't know until the ultrasound and blood tests. Tate stuck four pins in my head and a few in my arms and legs. The heated bed felt super nice since my feet were burning up from the lamp heater, which was moved during my midway check. It was one of the most soothing sessions I ever had. The pins in my head did wonders to calm my mind down.

Tate sent me home with a seven-day tincture that helped to keep everything in my tummy area "lifted." The Post-it attached to the bottle had some notes jotted down: pineapple, no lifting, soup, tincture for seven days.

The cramping increased during the evening and came with bright red bleeding every couple of hours. I was miscarrying by now, right? Essentially, it felt like I was having a period. I went into my pregnancy app, and it showed that my baby was the size of a blueberry. How cute. I entered the rabbit hole of community conversations and read about how some women bled bright red and still had healthy babies. That gave me some hope. The more I read the word "miscarriage," the more triggering it became. The anxiety was utterly exhausting.

After bleeding for a day and a half, I noticed that the bleeding occurred less frequently—a teaspoon every five hours or so. I felt so much better, and my mood was brighter. The cramping had subsided to a sporadically dull twinge. Did my body already get rid of what was living? I had no clue. I did a pregnancy test anyway to see if the line would be fainter than usual. It still came out brilliant, so I thought I would repeat it the next day. Since I still had a positive test, I told Micah I wanted to share the news with his family the next day, which was the family Christmas celebration. He didn't think it was a good idea since we still were unsure. We googled how long HCG (the pregnancy hormone) would stay within the system after a miscarriage. HCG can remain in your body for a few weeks despite steadily declining. It depends on the individual and how long they have been pregnant. I wanted to celebrate on a happy note, even though we were not 100% sure I was still pregnant. And, if I did have a miscarriage, I would at least have some support and understanding, whereas if we just gave the news of a lost baby, there would be only negative news. I want to be happy and celebrate that I was even able to become pregnant.

Despite trying to get pregnant for three and a half years and then finally becoming pregnant naturally, I couldn't even be joyous about any of it. It was a disappointment to be still cautious about every single bloody step! We talked some more and finally decided to tell the family with a disclaimer that it was still early and we hadn't had the first ultrasound yet. Realistically, I could very well be pregnant still, but we just weren't 100% positive, even with a 100% positive at-home test.

7. The Announcement

The morning before Micah's family Christmas gathering, I wanted to backtrack on the announcement because fear got hold of me. Maybe I wasn't pregnant any longer. I also didn't want to go anymore because I felt sad. We discussed it briefly and then decided to announce it with the caveat that I had a scare that week. We gathered everyone for a fake family photo, and Micah pretended to get ready to take a picture. He hit the record button and told everyone to say, "Juju's pregnant!"

I was directly in the center and felt the room fill with excitement. After the energy decreased a bit, both Micah and I told everyone that it was still quite early. We hadn't even had our first ultrasound, and we had a scare that week, so we hoped everything was going to be okay. One of Micah's sisters piped up and mentioned that she bled through most of her second child's pregnancy. Her husband tried hushing her "gross" story, but I explained that I needed this info and thanked her. Her two daughters ewwed at all of the details provided by their mother about her pregnancies and the miscarriage between the two. I appreciated the story and thought it was so important for women to share their experiences all the time, whether good or bad. Truly, I had no idea what I was going through and needed all of the information I could get.

Micah's brother noted how nourishing I looked. Did he mean nurturing? I knew he only meant well by this comment, but why did women need to look nurturing at all, and why is it that when some people find out you're pregnant, you suddenly look "motherly?" Just because I didn't want to hold and play with other people's kids every time I saw them doesn't mean I am not naturally nurturing. I was slightly offended because I didn't care for the labels society placed on women just because of their reproductive abilities. It was archaic and patriarchal. Micah thought it preposterous that I even felt this way because his brother said it; he meant it in a positive manner. However, as a woman and an individual, it was my right to feel how I felt. Was I not allowed to resist a "compliment" towards me? Did women always have to nod and smile like a Stepford wife?

During our continued conversations about the pregnancy, I let everyone know I was pregnant during Thanksgiving and was completely unaware as I took the pregnancy test a couple of days after the gathering. Micah's brother exclaimed, "I knew it!" Lol! This guy.

My schedule of bleeding that week was as follows:

Wednesday during sex and then before midnight.

Thursday and Friday, about two teaspoons every few hours.

Saturday, one teaspoon every five hours.

No blood until late Sunday afternoon. There was cramping and a coagulated blob with maybe another teaspoon later that night.

I took a couple more pregnancy tests, and both were positive, so I decided to wait another couple of days to retake them. I didn't feel bloaty in the morning, but I was when evening came. I was not nauseous but quite tired. I had no idea what was happening with my body; it was truly a mystery and was both frustrating and annoying. I googled what may have affected me negatively, i.e., certain foods and essential oils. Down another rabbit hole I went that drove me mad. I questioned if the tea I was drinking was detrimental or if any of the ingredients in my soup were deathly for my future baby. The madness was real. My mind spun uncontrollably.

Prego!!

On Christmas day, I wanted to surprise one of my best girlfriends, Vee, who had no clue about the anxiety I went through, as she had been going through her own shizzz lately. I handed her a Din Tai Fung paper bag, which was a very high-quality reusable bag. She opened it up, laughed at my other best girlfriend, S, and exclaimed, "Is this one of those prank gifts?" I was recording this charade, and the camera picked up everything, from when she laughed about getting pasta sauce to realizing that the label said Prego. I observed the wheels in her brain turning, clicking, and then realizing this was a pregnancy announcement. Vee immediately leaped off the couch to hug me, yelling, "Oh my god, you're pregnant!" She then predictably started to cry while S and I laughed at her. It was hilarious and sweet all at the same time. S already knew about my stressful week as she had come by two days after I started bleeding to catch up.

That evening, Micah handed the same bag to his sister, Panda. She looked up at him while seated on the couch and asked if he was pregnant.

8. The Ultrasound

I was a mix of emotions the morning of my ultrasound. It could go either way; my odds were fifty-fifty. I wanted to keep a logical hat on and be realistic about the situation. I did not want my emotions to get the best of me. I fear nothing regularly, but on that day, I feared losing a baby, which, for many women, was everything. To me, it was something, but not everything. I felt super lucky to have an incredibly loving and supportive husband, the cutest Shiba Inu for a pet, a terrific career, a side artist/modeling/acting career, wonderful girlfriends, a home to live in, food, water, internet, and The Witcher on Netflix. The most critical part was if I did miscarry, it at least meant that I could get pregnant naturally, which was something I thought would never occur. I was shivering inside with stress for one moment, then trying to calm my brain the next. What a rollercoaster.

I checked in, and the receptionist mumbled something so quickly that I barely heard it. All I heard was, "When you're ready." I overheard another lady check in, and the other receptionist told her to give a urine sample when she was ready. I then put two and two together and told the receptionist it was my first appointment. *Where do I go to give my sample?*

I was in the washroom, and there were directions on the wall. Wipe twice—once on the sides of the labia and then another wipe for the urethra area—then label the sample container. It took me five minutes to read the instructions for some reason, as I didn't want to do anything wrong. I was having a hard time concentrating. After almost fifteen minutes in there, I finally closed the metal door where the samples were collected.

Five minutes later, the receptionist called my name. Mari, the nurse's assistant, measured my height, weight, and blood pressure. During the health history updates, I let her know that I had some bleeding and thus wasn't sure if I was still pregnant. She continued her routine as if I was still pregnant. She left so I could undress and wait for Rita, the nurse practitioner, to do my ultrasound. I quickly got naked, put on the robe, placed the sheet over my lap, and put my phone right beside me just in case I was still pregnant and could take a video for Micah, who had to drive up north for some meetings.

Rita came in a few moments later. I heard her grab my chart from the slot right outside the door. She reintroduced herself to me, unaware that she had completed an ultrasound on me over a year ago, right before my first IUI. She mentioned that I had some bleeding, and that was when I lost it. I cried a bit. I usually do not cry easily. I told her that I was pretty nervous because of the bleeding. She handed me some tissues. She started with the ultrasound since she understood what I had gone through. The wand entered the opening of my vagina, and I watched the screen as Rita steered it in various directions. From my recollection of what I had seen of other ultrasounds early on in pregnancy, I realized that there was nothing but a black void. Rita confirmed my thoughts and pointed out a little blub that may still be floating around in my uterus. She noted that my left ovary produced a golden egg and commented that new follicles were growing, which was a good sign of my egg reserve. I still had eggs forming at the age of thirty-eight. Rita explained that right after week six, the clump of cells forming probably stopped, which then sent signals to halt HCG production, and that a zygote perhaps had not formed quite yet. When I was bleeding heavily at week seven, I had most likely miscarried a few days before that. At this point, I didn't feel sad or stressed out. I felt relief that I finally knew and could move on. My scientific logic came into place when Rita explained the intricacies to me.

Bloodbath

After I miscarried, I thought I was done bleeding for those four days. Wrong! I likely ovulated between days twelve and thirteen and started spotting again. We did have sex around that time since my body seemed like it was ready to go from the visions of the follicles via the ultrasound. I spotted for about five days, which then turned to heavier bleeding for four days, like I was on my period. I received a call from Rita, the NP, and she said my HCG levels were pretty high when I was tested. She told me to come in again to have another blood test. During this second round of bleeding, which was like a second miscarriage, my boobs were sore, and I was bloaty.

I was looking at my Instagram (IG) and saw a photo of Grimes—the awesome, super rad music artist from Canada—with her nipples and belly out. She had two different colored eyes and a fetus computer-generated onto her tummy. She looked cool, freaky, robot/alien-like. The nipple shot got taken down from IG as expected, and she posted the same photo with nipples edited out. The next day, Grimes had another photo that showed more of her growing tummy. I then had a whiny voice, thinking, why can Grimes have a baby and I can't? The way she lived her electronic robot Victorian lifestyle didn't even seem like she cared about having kids. But since I knew her so well (sarcasm), I thought I would judge from afar like a real, insecure human being. Micah commented on how skinny she looked in her "Violence" music video and thus was surprised when I shared with him Elon Musk was rumored to be the father. Don't get me wrong, I was thrilled to see Grimes preggy, but I was surprised this young woman, seven years younger than me, would have a baby before me. Her ovaries worked better than my geriatric ones. Sigh. I worked hard at getting pregnant and wanted that back. Like a crazed, unpredictable cat, I lashed out at anything I could get my claws on. Those thoughts were quite fleeting, but for the most part, I was fine.

I received a call from Rita, who notified me that my HCG level was now at four, which was reassuring. It also looked like my body was going back to normal. She assumed that I had more miscarriage tissue to get rid of and said my bleeding should taper off soon. I was relieved to hear this information but also sad again about the loss.

Micah wanted to have all of our ducks in a row, so he called the other big fertility clinic in Seattle to see if our insurance was accepted. The finance department sent an e-mail indicating that the wording from the insurance company seemed to contradict itself, but when she called, it looked like we would be covered.

9. Getting Back to Normal

It was a month after what I thought was the first day of my period. It was difficult to tell because it was the second round of bleeding after the miscarriage, which occurred within two weeks. I watched for the signs of ovulation, which seemed normal for this cycle. I noticed my body becoming slimmer and finally being less bloated. It felt good not to feel big, and because I am a petite Asian woman, you can tell if I gained any weight. My double-zero dresses stopped fitting me, and it sucked because I had so many. I felt thin for maybe a good week and a bit. Around days twenty to twenty-two, I felt weird, like I wasn't myself.

I remembered reading *Like a Mother: A Feminist Journey Through the Science and Culture of Pregnancy* by Angela Garbes, who, coincidentally, lived in Seattle. The book spoke about microchimerism, where the mother harbors fetal cells even after a miscarriage or abortion. In a January 2018 article titled "We are Multitudes" in the Aeon newsletter written by Katherine Rowland, Microchimera is Greek and translates to a fire-breathing monster with the head of a lion, a goat's body, and a serpent's tail. (https://aeon.co/essays/microchimerism-how-pregnancy-changes-the-mothers-very-dna)

I was feeling off because of the fetal cell remnants from my first pregnancy. My body felt alien to me, and I didn't know what to do about it. So, with each pregnancy, our bodies continue accumulating fetal cells, which can travel through the bloodstream and embed into different organs. These foreign cells continue to live inside you forever. Thus, you will always physically have a part of your child in you. My body was no longer wholly mine, and I wondered how it had been affected and what had evolved. According to researchers from the Cincinnati Children's Hospital, these cells were purposefully retained to ensure the genetic fitness of future offspring. So it was like each sibling was helping to promote a genetically sound environment for the next to ensure better survival and decrease risk of certain diseases.

So, day twenty-eight rolled by, and I was expecting my period. The nurse mentioned my period should come back in about four to six weeks. I continued to monitor and see how my body reacted. I noticed some pimples to the left of my neck and to the left of my chin that had formed. Maybe my hormones were trying to get back on track. Who knew? I noticed my tummy became bloated and sighed because my sense of being thinner had already dissipated. I had no other signs of getting my period except for the bloating.

On day thirty, it was a palindromic day – 02.02.2020. Wouldn't it be interesting to find out I was pregnant on this super neato numerical patterned day where one hasn't occurred in 909 years? So I took a pregnancy test and didn't see anything, but the faintest, faintest, skinniest blue line appeared after two minutes. I could even see the dye being slightly dragged out from the control. I was unsure what to think and didn't want to get my hopes up. I stowed the test in my top bathroom drawer. I re-checked it a few times, more closely examining it each time. If I were pregnant, it would have been too early to tell, and maybe implantation would have occurred later in my cycle, which was plausible. I decided to wait until the morning of 2.4.20 to take another test. Again, I saw a faint blue line that was slightly darker than the first test, but it was still not an entirely positive test. My boobs were now becoming somewhat sore, and I noticed slight lower abdominal tweaks. My exhaustion levels had been increasing, and I had been sneezing. Maybe those were my usual PMS symptoms presenting themselves? I suppose I would take another test the following day.

On a different side note—one worth mentioning—was the "controversy" with JLo and Shakira's Super Bowl halftime show, where delicate (older) non-BIPOC people were offended by two Latinas dancing skillfully on stage while singing. The attire was akin to stripper wear since JLo showed off her fabulous pole strength. Slut shaming comments were flagrantly thrown onto news and social media. Many women even addressed how the performance was a slap in the face to the #metoo moment, which was entirely idiotic, in my opinion. Truly, what was displayed during that halftime segment was women empowerment from a forty-three and fifty-year-old, both women of color. To say that this performance went against #metoo was feeding into the patriarchy and a continuation of rape culture. The notion that women deserved what they got for wearing skanky clothes was victim-blaming at its finest. The cherry on top was the children in cages to protest the horrendous practices of border control, ICE, and the pulling of immigrant families apart. There probably will never be another half-time show that implements powerful, moving messages and matriarchal symbolism.

Pregnancy Tests Can Add Up

The following day, I tested again with a different brand to see if I would get different results. The control popped up all brilliant, and I didn't see anything in the other circle, so I concluded I was not pregnant. I hung on to the stick anyway and thought I saw a faint line, but it seemed inconclusive. Hoping, waiting, and wishing were so exhausting. Micah thought I was testing too early. So I waited a whole day, tested again, and saw a faint line, although this one was slightly darker than the last test. My boobs were still sore, and the next morning, I felt some extreme, twingy cramping in my abdomen. I imagined a little ball of multiplying cells trying to burrow itself further into my womb. My intuition told me this was me being pregnant. I was on my third box of tests—going through them like water—and tested in the afternoon. I saw two lines indicating a positive test; one line was slightly lighter, but the test was positive. I told Micah, "Happy belated."

Saturday arrived. We had dinner plans with one of my best girlfriends and her French lover. I wanted to surprise her with the news and asked Micah what he thought.

"Well, it's up to you, but I would wait," Micah said.

"You want me to wait until after my first trimester? That's so long! You know, people lose their babies after three months, even at six months! If I wait and then have another miscarriage, then I will be sharing sad news with my friends or going through it alone."

"Alone? I am here."

"I know, honey, but it isn't the same. It's good to get support from other women, especially those who know what I am going through."

"Hmm ya, I see that. Either way, it is ultimately up to you."

"But you wouldn't tell anyone yet?"

"I wouldn't, but it's your decision, and I support it."

I found it funny that we were having this conversation again, with the same dialogue and thought process. Maybe Micah thought that if we lost it again, we wouldn't have to tell anyone, but to me, that was the recipe for bouts of depression and lack of support. I needed as much support and love as possible; while my partner could be there for me, I needed more than that. Part of the grieving and healing process was me telling my story, being okay to tell it, and moving on from it. I have witnessed the result of internalizing traumatic situations. The biggest delusion that erupted was the belief that we are totally fine when we are not.

Micah and I went back and forth a little more, and I saw the wheels turning in his head as he came to the same understanding as when we first had this conversation in December before Christmas. I, too, was fearful that if I shared with our closest friends and family, I would miscarry again, and it would be a just kidding moment. By the way, I could barely type that last sentence because it frightened me even to type "miscarry." Wow, PTSD at its finest. The duality of my feelings reminded me of the duality of my zodiac sign. I was happy yet scared. The astonishment of becoming pregnant directly after my first miscarriage created an electrical energy in my aura. Unfortunately, fear usually won, but I loved surprising my girlfriends with every chance I got. So, after we agreed that it was okay to share our news with our closest friends and family, I went upstairs to see how I could present my pee stick as a bamboozle. I found the best thing ever! A Neiman Marcus gift box!

We had a reservation at Musang, this cute Filipino bistro. I handed over the fancy box after ordering our drinks (mine was non-alcoholic; I don't usually drink).

"Oh, maybe it's a sex toy?" my silly, fiery girlfriend said to her French lover, who started to slide the ribbon off the box. He opened the package and kind of stared at it for a bit. They both finally realized what it was, were overcome with excitement, and got up to hug us.

Nervously and giddily, I chimed in, "It is still very early, but I wanted to share this because it happened so fast after the first one. Hopefully, this one sticks. I guess my body is telling me okay, we are ready now."

Micah added, "Oh, and we are getting a Shiba Inu puppy too."

We had an appointment the next morning to see the puppies, who were just over a week old. When it rains, it pours babies—literally.

Don't Be Afraid to Share

People love to tell others how to go about announcing their pregnancy and to keep mum about the miscarriage. I admit I also had my opinions as well before I ever got pregnant. It used to be an old practice back in the day to wait until after the first trimester to share news of the pregnancy to the world; miscarriages were more common in the 1800s. One of my friends shared her news just a couple of days after testing positive, and I judged her for telling everyone so soon because I believed she should have waited. What did I know back then? Unfortunately, she ended up miscarrying right after her first trimester. Her mother told her she was not to speak of her miscarriage outwardly to save face, which was so old-school Asian culture. After having my own experiences, I felt that telling those closest to me was necessary so they could be there for me, for good or bad. Being able to verbalize my loss was part of the healing process and could be cathartic.

10. Can I Be Happy Now?

It was four days after Valentine's Day in 2020, and I had been having difficulty being happy for this new baby. I wanted to be realistic that things could go wrong at any moment. I kept saying things like, "Hopefully, this one sticks," or "We'll see what happens." What didn't help was the nurse calling me back today and telling me that my HCG levels increased a bit, but they didn't double, which was what should have occurred within forty-eight hours. She advised me to take another blood test next Monday. I texted a couple of my closest girlfriends who tried to comfort me, tell me not to worry or stress, and not look at the internet. Too late. I googled "slowly rising HCG levels," and ectopic pregnancy and miscarriage were the top hits. Hmm, wonderful. I read about ectopic pregnancy briefly and dismissed that diagnosis since I didn't have any pelvic pain, plus I did feel the embryo burrowing into me early on. Maybe this baby wanted to develop slowly? Micah then wondered if his spermies were to blame since his first wife also had a miscarriage, and I said yes right away because I had been working super hard at getting pregnant while he didn't modify any lifestyle changes. Truly, it was frustrating to invest so much of myself when there was another part to the equation, and it wasn't just about the bloody golden egg! Sperm needs to be of high quality, too, and this was what society needed to understand: that it wasn't just about the woman and her fertility capabilities. Men provide 50% of their DNA to the zygote!

<u>Waiting Game</u>

Yesterday, I went to the lab for the third time to get my HCG blood work completed. The tech, of course, recognized me, and while I sat in the blood draw chair, she told me how her weekend was, which consisted of dealing with her alcoholic husband, who hit rock bottom again. I responded with concern and empathy while sharing that my ex had drug addiction problems. She added that her husband's brother and father also had addiction problems; thus, it ran in the family. It wasn't the experience I expected this time, but at least it took my mind off worrying for a tiny bit.

Throughout the day, I continued to remind myself that it would be okay if my results weren't positive. Micah mentioned that maybe we should consider IVF in the next round. I was always a proponent of "third time's the charm!" Since this was the second time, there was always hope. Truly, we felt time was ticking away, and we didn't want to miss our chances of having healthy children.

My girlfriends were so sweet, texting me and asking if I was okay. I was wondering if I had received my results yet. It was no fun waiting and worrying, but having friends to offer their love and support was the sun, moon, and stars.

I got a call before 1 pm, and the caller ID showed Seattle OBGYN. I got nervous.

"Hello?" I answered.

"Hi Juliet, it's Seattle OBGYN. Do you have a moment to speak?"

"Ummm…"

"It's nothing scary, so there's no need to worry."

"Oh, okay."

"Looks like your HCG levels did increase. They are just over 1,000; they were at 141 the last time. Typically, we see a value of about 3000 at this stage, but either way, this increase is a positive sign. We want to schedule an ultrasound with you next week."

"I already have one scheduled for Monday."

"Oh yes, let me double check… perfect. Everything is set!"

"Great! So, I believe I am still pretty early in the pregnancy, but it is hard to tell because I wasn't sure when my period started. I had two rounds of bleeding, and I believe I ovulated two weeks after I stopped bleeding. I do think that I had implantation much later in my cycle. And I was speaking to my acupuncturist, who mentioned that I could have ovulated twice. Is that possible?"

"It sounds like after you miscarried, you didn't have your period and got pregnant right away, so it is possible that you just ovulated much later on, which I think is truly the case."

"Oh, interesting. Okay, well, thank you so much for all the info."

"You're welcome! We'll see you next week."

"Thank you, bye!"

I was so relieved when I heard her say, "It's nothing scary." This new info about how I never had a period was quite intriguing. I was about to text my girlfriends and realized that I had to tell the father of my baby first. Micah was like, "What? You didn't have your period?"

I was like, "I know, crazy, right?" This concept was so novel to us that it caused multiple mind explosions. I wrote to my girlfriends that I had good news, but of course, we still had to wait for the ultrasound to ensure things were progressing appropriately. Also, if I were earlier than eight weeks along, there was a chance the heartbeat would not be present just yet. So now, I had another thing to worry about, but at least I had some good news.

Intro to Pregnancy

It was now the end of February. We attended this intro pregnancy class at the OBGYN office. We were handed a folder that was clearly printed by Amazon, noting how easy it was to create a registry with them. By the way, I do not care for Amazon at all. We don't have Prime and will never subscribe unless the warehouse workers have better working conditions and higher wages. Even the corporate office employees are treated horribly. I know because my friends have worked there; one close girlfriend still does. I have no clue why she thinks she needs to continue tormenting herself. Maybe the enduring, Chinese hard worker in her believes she must suffer to get a massive payoff. The payoff, unfortunately, will be a ton of therapy bills due to uncontrollable anxiety and stress. Anyhow, Amazon had infiltrated this OBGYN office, and I was disgusted.

We sat in the waiting room with just one other couple. It seemed like it was going to be a very small class. At a quarter past five, a nurse manager came in and introduced herself. She was a middle-aged woman with a blonde bob hairstyle. Her manner of speaking told me she had done this intro class too many times, but was still very enthusiastic. She went through all of the content in the packet, and this was what I got out of it:

Insurance didn't cover everything, i.e., certain genetic testing and the number of ultrasounds (there was one that cost more than $2K. I had hopes that Bernie Sanders would win the presidential campaign so we could finally have universal healthcare).

It was rare, but you could get Listeria from unpasteurized cheese and deli meats. However, heating and cooking them killed off the bacteria. Big fish contained lots of mercury.

Influenza and Tdap (prevents whooping cough) vaccines are recommended, and the people who visit your baby must be up-to-date with these vaccines, too. (Micah's father didn't believe in the flu vaccine. I guess he won't see the baby for a while.)

Sex was okay. (I am going to come back to this one.)

No raw sushi.

Micah asked why pregnant women's immune systems were so fragile. We learned it was to protect the baby and ensure that the mom's immune system wasn't harming the baby and thinking it was a foreign invader (even though it was a parasite, as per my Biology 101 textbooks).

It was great to do these classes as a couple so we'd be informed and on the same page. It also provided a bonding experience between both of us and the baby. The shared responsibility became more apparent.

11. You Want to Do What?

Today, Micah was being extra lovey with me and told me he wanted to fool around. I was like, "Oh, ya? Good story, honey." We hadn't had sex in maybe three weeks or so, but Micah's second brain thought it had been three months. Truly, I had been trying to keep my body as stress-free as possible, and the last time I was pregnant and we had sex, I bled and then miscarried. So I had PTSD from that experience, and even seeing the color red or even something as simple as drinking from a red-coloured cup triggered me. It was wild and nerve-wracking.

Throughout the day, Micah flirted and cuddled with me to let me know he missed my body. We took our little Shiba bear for a walk, and he mentioned how, when we got home, we should go upstairs and pleasure each other. I told him I still had work, and he sulked a bit. Micah went upstairs to rest when we returned, and I sat on the couch to do more work. I got a call from my girlfriend, and I started gabbing loudly. I noticed a new text from Micah.

Micah: *I thought you were working?*

Me: *I didn't know she was going to call me.*

After I got off the phone, I received another text.

Micah: *I miss you.*

I got up, grabbed some hot water, and went upstairs. I knew what Micah wanted, but I wasn't in the mood. I got to the bedroom, and he was lying in bed with his eyes open.

"Hi, honey. Why do you miss me so much?" I asked.

"Because I do, and I want to be close to you," Micah said.

I got into bed and lay down next to him. "Well, I didn't know I was going to get a call, and I haven't spoken to her in a while."

"You know we haven't had sex in a while."

"You got some like three days ago, and you want more?"

"Well, I can't help if I want to have sex with my wife like every day!"

"You know I am scared of losing the baby, and I have PTSD from the miscarriage. So these feelings do not make me want to have sex."

"Well, the nurse in the class said it was okay to have sex."

"Ya, that still doesn't make me feel less triggered! You know you're being selfish, right? I am being entirely selfless with this baby and ensuring I am careful with my body."

"Well, what do you want me to do? You want me to go and find someone to have sex with? I physically need to be close to you! I don't want to masturbate; that's boring and stupid! Even when I was masturbating daily, I still wanted to have sex with you. I would have sex with you twice a day if I could!"

We went back and forth more, and then I said we could cuddle. But cuddling always led to more, and Micah started removing my clothes. After a little while, I gave in and thought, well, if the nurse said it was okay, I guess it was all right. Micah made sure to be as gentle as possible, and there wasn't any blood, thank goodness.

Later that night, I spoke with my girlfriend, Lena. She also had a miscarriage, but now, being over forty, she has a beautiful and healthy seven-month-old. We chatted about "geriatric" ovaries and how hard it was for older moms. She mentioned that she told her husband that there would be no sex for the first trimester and highly advised that I do the same, as uterine contractions may occur during sex.

I, of course, started googling about sex during the first trimester, and most of the posts said sex was safe in a healthy pregnancy. There didn't seem to be any studies referencing this notion. I found one opinion piece that stated doctors should be careful when saying sex is safe for all pregnancies at any time during the pregnancy, since each case is different. Also, there had been no studies completed to indicate that sex was safe for all pregnancies. I told Micah that I felt anxiety about having sex in the first trimester, and that was all he needed to hear.

Speaking about sex, from various online sources/groups, I noticed a trend in how some women are quite upset about their partners' porn viewing. For example, the wife finds out about the husband's secret porn use, and he thinks it's no biggie. However, he continues to lie about it, and she feels it's a form of infidelity and damages emotional intimacy. The trust has been eroded.

I notice a few issues here in general. The first issue is that the husband lied to his wife, which eroded trust within the relationship. One husband's remark was, "All guys watch porn," which is such a scapegoat that lacks accountability. The second issue is if these husbands are masturbating and not taking care of their wives' sexual needs, then there is intimate selfishness, which is a step towards complacency. Plus, these wives may even feel rejected in bed because the husbands have already satisfied themselves and are no longer interested. If these men were to put away their devices, turn off the porn, and have an actual intimate moment with their wives in real life instead of their hands, they would have felt more secure (and satisfied) in general. Porn is being seen as the mistress because it's literally taking the husband away. What a waste of time and energy to fawn over digital imagery.

Nurturing one's partnership takes work, and it isn't difficult, nor should it be. Truly, love is pretty simple. You need to put in the effort. If women don't feel heard, their feelings aren't validated, AND there hasn't been an orgasm in a long time—there will be consequences. Plus, there are other gentlemen who would be more than willing to. Just sayin'.

When I was with my ex, I had huge issues with him going to see strippers. Maybe I was insecure at that age, or perhaps he didn't make me feel secure enough. In essence, I wasn't being appropriately satisfied, and he was off happily pleasuring himself to some porn instead. Eventually, I fell out of love with him. With Micah, I never cared if he watched porn because I was super secure with our love, and he was responsible for creating this nurturing environment. I didn't even care too much if he occasionally went to the strip club. I think the only time I had an issue was during my first pregnancy, and we were in Vegas. I had to go on a work trip, and Micah tagged along. He was bored one evening and thought we should watch strippers. I was not too fond of the idea at that time. Maybe it was the pregnancy hormones, but I didn't want my husband to go to a strip club while I was carrying his child. He respected that and was fine with not going.

Telltale Signs

I ordered the sweetest Fair Isle Christmas sweater when I first got pregnant. It was for three to six months, and it would have been the perfect timing if I had been still pregnant with that one. After a few weeks, I noticed it wasn't delivered yet and contacted the store. They gave me a refund and said it still may show up. Well, it did, two months later. I took it as a sign that this second pregnancy was a keeper, and this sweater would still be perfect even if it fit after Christmas.

The Night Before the Ultrasound

I had been having a brown discharge the past three or four days, which initially seemed to alarm my acupuncturist, but she quickly brushed it off, saying everything was fine. It was most likely a quick turn in reaction so as not to stir my anxiety. That Sunday afternoon, I saw brighter red spots of blood. At first, I thought maybe it was normal. It occurred again later that night with a tiny cramp, and then right before bed, a large glob had ejected itself from me. I tried not to freak the eff out. Everything will be fine, I told myself.

The next morning, we headed to the OBGYN appointment. A lady came in and told me she was a physician's assistant (PA) and would be doing my ultrasound. I let her know that I had some bleeding, so she decided that we should begin with the ultrasound. I got nervous and hoped that something, anything but an empty womb, would pop up on the screen. The wand was placed into the opening of my vagina and maneuvered around a bit until a small circle popped up. The PA said she saw the fetal stalk, and it looked like I was just over five weeks, which seemed a bit inaccurate to me. She measured the circle's dimensions and printed a screenshot for us to take home. She told us to come back in a week for a viability check, and if I started bleeding a bunch, there was no need to come in since it would most likely be a miscarriage.

This was like a recurring nightmare. The feeling of helplessness was unmanageable. I want my body to do what I thought it should be doing since the day my DNA decided I would have ovaries. Having easy, healthy pregnancies was society's assumption of our wombs. This sentiment was engrained very early on, and girls are not educated that the outcome could become a nightmare. Sex education should be an entire course on its own, not a one-hour session with barely enough time for Q&A. Why was it still so taboo for school? I mean, I have a few thoughts, i.e., patriarchy, religion, and right-wing politics. The more information girls have about their bodies, the better they can navigate their reproductive evolution. There would be fewer unexpected or unwanted pregnancies, more control over one's body, and healthier women in general.

I probably already knew that my body was doing a repeat of the first miscarriage. It was scary yet no longer unfamiliar, unfortunately. There was a feeling of defeat, sadness, and longing for hope. All in all, Micah and I were grateful for the little blurry screenshot of our embryo, even if it was possible that it would not be viable by next week. The silver lining still glowed for us.

12. Super Tuesday 2020

It was a head-to-head battle between Bernie Sanders and Joe Biden for the democratic debate. Micah was a nervous wreck because he knew Sanders would be screwed over somehow. That afternoon, I saw more bleeding. I tried not to freak out, but then, when it came at regular intervals with more gushing combined with cramping, I knew it was over. Micah and I comforted each other best, but we were both disappointed. Somehow, hope still lingered. The following day, I got up and started working as usual, as if it were another typical day. I had two presentations to prepare for the next day; thus, taking a sick day to grieve my loss was not an option. This was the life of a career woman. I had my second miscarriage, and I carried on presenting scientific data on influenza vaccines as if my womb wasn't suffering—as if I wasn't suffering. Yes, I could have taken the time off, but I didn't see the point then. Perhaps I needed the distraction from fertility realities. Also, I was excellent at my job, and thus, I forged on like an enduring lady boss. I did not cry and, therefore, surmised that I was doing all right.

That morning, Micah mentioned the night before sucked because of the miscarriage and because Biden astonishingly won more states than Sanders. Politics was so rigged. Fertility was so crushing.

What is That?

It was my third day of heavy bleeding, and we were out for dinner at a fantastic French bistro with friends. Dessert was about to arrive, and I felt more intense cramping. A gush of blood came out. When we finally got home, I changed my pad, and literally, one minute later, I felt another gush of blood, so I got back into the bathroom to see if I needed to change pads again. What I saw was something I had never seen before. It was the little embryo fully intact with a long, thin cord attached, which I assumed was the umbilical cord. I was about to toss my findings into the toilet when I placed it on some toilet paper and inspected it. The embryo was a deep red sac, probably smaller than my thumb. I poked at it with my fingernail and noticed that it had the consistency of a soft rubber ball, almost in the shape of a human heart. I was curious to see if it had a smell and put my nose close to it. I was amazed that it smelled earthy, like a fresh garden, in the evening. I kept smelling it to see if I was hallucinating, but it smelled nice and sweet, which to me seemed extremely bizarre, as it was basically a ball of dead cells and blood. I realized that I couldn't just flush it down the toilet. I felt terrible for the little thing.

"Honey, you want to see it?"

"What? No."

"Are you sure? It's really cool."

Micah came upstairs, and we both stared at it. He seemed intrigued for a few moments. I decided to cremate the little fetus. I grabbed a tin that was holding an old, large candle and tore up a bunch of paper from the recycling bin to act as kindling. I went out onto our tiny little patio and started lighting up matches. It took me about five matches to finally get anything started. I wanted to watch it burn, but too much smoke was building up, so I went inside and watched behind the sliding glass doors. Micah came over and was like what the heck are you doing? He shook his head at the smoke collecting at the top of our patio, probably seeping into our house.

Other Options?

I was at the OBGYN office again. The midwife came in a few minutes after the assistant and introduced herself.

"So let's see how far along your baby is coming and make sure it is growing properly."

"What? Did my notes not get updated? I just told the assistant who took my blood pressure that I miscarried last week, so this appointment is to check that everything has ejected itself."

45

I was flabbergasted and then had to retell my story again to the midwife, which was annoying and upsetting.

I wasn't emotional until the midwife started being sympathetic towards me. Micah mentioned that he also started feeling sorry for us at this very moment. Great, so now my husband was pitying our situation. In general, the appointment was informative; the ultrasound showed that the embryo had fully come out of my body, and the nurse advised us to wait until my next full period to try again, which may take some time to recalibrate and get on track. In my head, I was like, was there time for me to "wait" another cycle? Yes, I had girlfriends who had children over forty, but I was not taking any chances at this rate. I thought it was pretty miraculous that I became pregnant soon after my first miscarriage. Perhaps my body needed a rest, but I felt like the clock was ticking at the speed of light!

We were told that there was about a twenty-five percent chance of miscarriage on the first pregnancy. After a second miscarriage, this risk increased to thirty to forty percent, and after a third pregnancy, my chances of miscarriage could reach seventy-five percent. These statistics made me feel ill and that I should give up. Micah thought we should do IVF straight away. I was willing to take my chances on a third pregnancy if it occurred soon after, but I agreed there was no time to waste.

13. Aloha COVID-19

We were Hawaii-bound the very week the coronavirus made its spectacular mass spread in the US. Changes to health policy, work policy, and even mundane routines like going to Costco or getting a coffee were being restricted on the daily as new cases and deaths increased. My company went from "please be careful while traveling" to "no travel to China," to "only travel within your country," to "if you are uncomfortable with traveling, please speak with your manager." Essentially, Skype and phone calls became the primary forms of communication for meetings. Social distancing was now the biggest buzz term of the year, which brought on a thicker, palpable tension than what was emitted during the democratic primaries on social media. One side of the fence was the "shame on you for not isolating at home and risking the lives of others due to selfish boredom," while the opposing party was like, "I am young and so carefree and will never die, and I don't care about anyone else." So many fingers were pointing at each other, which led to more hostility and volatility. The divisiveness was as tall as the walls at the US-Mexico border.

Washington was the first state to have an epidemic that began in a nursing home in the city of Kirkland, a twenty-five-minute drive from my house. Schools and restaurants shut down just a couple of days after we departed for Kona. This trip was planned back a few months ago, and I had gone through two miscarriages literally within two months of each other. My well-being would be on the line if I didn't take a vacation. We did feel slightly guilty about being in a beautiful, warm spot while everyone was fighting for the last roll of toilet paper on the shelves during the lockdown. Seattle folks became hoarders within a week; it was unnecessary and greedy. After a few days, we realized that isolating ourselves was pretty simple on an island where we knew nobody. Sheltering in place never felt so good. The other thing we hoped was that we didn't bring COVID-19 onto the island.

I was sick with a head cold and dry cough, but no fever, chills, muscle aches, or shortness of breath. However, I never could be sure if I did have it as I was never tested. And there was no way I would be tested because I was not exhibiting all of the symptoms. The US had a shortage of COVID-19 tests. People were tested if they were intubated. During this pandemic, it was so telling that the healthcare system failed. There was a lack of protective equipment such as N95 masks, hospital gowns and beds, respirators, and even healthcare professionals. Healthcare coverage in the US was not socialized like in Canada and other European nations. Thus, many poor or uninsured people died without proper care. Despite being the world's most influential and prosperous country, America could not adequately protect its citizens.

Maybe it was my age and my type O blood that made me more resilient to the virus. Who knew? I mean, I did have a couple of miscarriages, and my body was probably trying its darndest to get back to normal. I blamed Micah for getting me sick as he fell ill before me; however, it only lasted for a couple of days.

I had one girlfriend ask me if my trip was previously planned and not just some whim to take advantage of super low flight rates (she had no clue about what I was going through, but even if she did, she's one who goes by the books). As she was a healthcare professional, I felt her judgment and noticed she kept posting about proper social distancing techniques on her FB and IG. Mind you, I agreed with all of those posts, and I thought folks needed to be responsible for keeping high-risk individuals safe and not continuing to spread the virus. I am a scientist, and my PhD dissertation was on viral infections, specifically HPV, and I understood the impact of proper precautions and preventative measures. The vast majority do not understand that there was no prior immunity to coronavirus; thus, no treatment or vaccine is available for a highly contagious microorganism. Besides taking a couple of plane rides, I felt we were being as responsible as possible in distancing ourselves. I was trying to do "my part" on my social media in spreading (pun not intended) news on COVID-19 and how serious it was. It was astonishing that some people were not taking this seriously enough. There were still so many unknowns, but the Centers for Disease Control and Prevention (CDC) was doing its best (hopefully).

On March 22nd, 2020, we were still about a week behind the disaster Italy was facing. The virus hit them so hard that their healthcare infrastructure was unable to handle such a high amount of severe cases. If we weren't prepared, this could be the exact pandemic scenario for the US. Truly, it was only the end of the beginning. (I've always wanted to say that; it sounds so profoundly detrimental.)

No IVF for You!

One of my girlfriends told me that her sister was finally considering freezing her eggs, and then she sent her an article on how COVID-19 was affecting reproductive medicine policies. In essence, there would be no new IVF procedures or other fertility assistance procedures until further notice. Micah and I were quite upset about this news. My appointment with the new fertility clinic, the one that accepted my insurance, was on the 31st of March. There was a possibility things would change, but at the time, there was very little data as to whether COVID-19 was harmful to pregnancies. So far, what I had read was that there hadn't been any issues with newborns whose mothers tested positive for COVID-19, but it was still too early for definitive answers. My ovaries went into panic mode when I was googling. It was best not to stress, but this new virus was ruining everyone's lives. It was ubiquitous.

April Showers Bring May Flowers?

The COVID-19 shelter-in-place/lockdown policy was still in place until the end of April for the state of Washington. Many were trying their hardest not to crack, resisting the ever-so-tempting urge to make plans with their friends. Even Micah wondered if we could see our friends in an outdoor spot, poor thing. Everyone missed eating out, having a drink with buddies, and not having to sanitize their hands every two minutes. I was sure parents were tired of homeschooling, disciplining, feeding, and caring for their kids while working from home. Those living paycheck-to-paycheck, who no longer had a job and still had to pay their rent and bills, were the ones I worried about the most. Even more horrifying, those who had to shelter-in-place with their domestic abuser. The world had become scarier, even depressing, and no end was in sight.

There were social media posts about how if you weren't productive during this pandemic by learning a new skill or starting some side hustle with all of the newly found time you had, you basically sucked. I wondered what burnt-out parents thought about this statement. On the other hand, some articles said you needed to ignore these "productive" posts and get through this chaos alive. Mentally speaking, people may not have been doing well. Grief, anxiety, depression, restlessness, and lack of sleep were some of the issues many faced. I had a feeling virtual therapy was quite lucrative those days.

For the past month, I felt hopeless. Two miscarriages and a pandemic could stir up some anxious feelings. At the end of March, we had a virtual meeting with the fertility doctor at Seattle Reproductive Medicine (SRM). She was very empathetic, knowledgeable, and truly understood our situation. This first meeting left me with a feeling of renewed hope and relief. We were told that our situation would deem our fertility services "essential" and that we could probably start a round of IVF when I got my next cycle. I thought all was lost during this state of isolation and lockdown, but because of the "essential" category, I may have my COVID baby after all.

The option of genetic testing of the embryos was discussed at great length. The issue here was if I did not have many viable eggs, with the attrition rate so high, there was the possibility of losing embryos. Essentially, with each step of the IVF process, i.e., egg collection, sperm insertion, embryo growth, and genetic testing, viability was at high risk. The process may be limited if I didn't have many viable eggs. The hope was after proper embryo growth. I would have at least a few healthy-looking ones to implant. If I miraculously had twenty fetched eggs, I would be golden, but beggars couldn't be choosers at my age. The thing I was most fearful of was not having any viable eggs.

I spoke to one of my graduate schoolmates who recently had a set of twins. She and her wife went through more than two years of fertility assistance, ranging from multiple rounds of IUI to two rounds of IVF. The first round of IVF resulted in no viable eggs, so they decided to adopt two embryos. Embryo adoption IVF was much cheaper than regular IVF and cheaper/easier than regular adoption.

Micah and I spoke about whether embryo adoption was something we would consider, and that was a short conversation. At that moment, we did not wish to raise kids that we did not produce. Was that narcissistic of us? Perhaps it could be seen that way, but we preferred to merge our DNA and have this be a real-life representation of our love. And, if it ended up that we couldn't have kids, we may be DINKs for life with fur babies.

14. Cycle Day Two

It was April 5th, 2020, and I just started my cycle, which had been on sabbatical for over four months. I called SRM in the morning and spoke with my advising nurse, who had to get a little caught up with the urgency of my case and the "essential" status that our doctor bestowed upon us. She gave us a checklist of what we needed from our last fertility clinic, i.e., blood lab work, hormone level results, etc. We frantically signed consent forms, took screenshots of our lab results in the meantime, and gave someone my credit card number to pay $15K up front because my insurance had to go through some pre-authorizations first, which apparently would take a couple of weeks, and then had another virtual call with our doctor, who I will now refer to as Dr. Bird because she reminded me of Wendy Byrd from the Ozark show.

Quite a bit of pertinent info was thrown at us in a very organized fashion. I appreciated the urgency the doctor and her team felt for this upcoming cycle being the one to start. I did not feel any urgency from the last clinic and had to push for things to get done. Dr. Bird actively listened to me and then deciphered what was best for my situation. When shopping around for a fertility doctor, I think this was a deal breaker or maker—that the doctor fully understands what you want and tries to incorporate that into the procedure and practice as best as possible. I felt like our doctor gave us options and spoke about the risks and benefits of each. Thus, her guidance was paramount in our decision-making. Dr. Bird was optimistic yet realistic at the same time.

Dr. Bird asked us again if we were okay with the prospect of having twins if we only had two viable embryos, and that if this were the case, we would be doing a transfer into my uterus at day three of growth. This option of having a transfer on day three was surprising to me because I had always thought the embryos were supposed to grow for at least five days. Essentially, what I learned was the longer you waited for the embryos to grow, the higher the chances of losing more viable ones. So, there was loss with each stage and with time, and Dr. Bird wanted to salvage as much as possible. We were okay with twins since we would get more bang for our buck, and we were running out of time. So, two birds, one stone, ya? Dr. Bird thought that with my hormone levels, I might be able to get two to five viable eggs. I hoped I could at least get that. My worst fear was that I wouldn't have any quality eggs. Sigh, women are so hard on themselves.

I got a call in the afternoon from the clinic's finance department. My insurance no longer needed pre-authorizations, so I got my $15K back and only had to pay $1,599. This was astonishing and wonderful news. I would have likely been refunded after the insurance was approved, but it was nice not to have to dish out an enormous amount of money upfront.

I received a calendar from the nurse with the planned IVF cycle. On the 2nd day of my cycle, I needed to begin birth control pills as this aided in preparing my ovaries for stimulation. I looked at when I would possibly have the embryo transfer, and if everything went as planned, this would occur as soon as possible on April 27th! I was shocked that I may be pregnant in just another month. I scheduled a suppression check ultrasound appointment for Friday, when I also had to do an office hysteroscopy where they would stick a tiny camera up my cervix and look to see if my uterus was kosher.

Liquid Gold

I got a phone call from the fertility pharmacy, and they listed all the meds I was to receive. I just agreed because I had no idea what Dr. Bird prescribed for me. The pharmacist went through how much I owed out of pocket, which came out to just over $1,800. Well, there went the majority of my Health Savings Account (HSA) funds. I then asked how much my insurance covered, which was over 10K! I was wondering now if I just blew through my IVF insurance coverage or if I had a separate prescription amount that was covered as well. I would assume I had already spent $10K worth of IVF coverage.

The package came the next day, as it should have if you had spent that kind of money. The most expensive part was the Gonal, which was around $800 a pop; I needed eight boxes. I was told an abundant supply of breast milk was liquid gold. Truly, hormone juice in a syringe was much more lucrative. I need to purchase some stocks in fertility pharma.

The More, the Merrier

I had my first in-person visit to the fertility clinic. They had to do a COVID-19 screening with a fever check, and I needed to wear a mask. Micah wasn't allowed to enter. I was asked to come in with a full bladder, and I already needed to go to the washroom. I took 400mg of ibuprofen, which was half of what they suggested for the procedures that were about to occur (my system is sensitive to meds).

Unsurprisingly, the waiting room was sparse, but the three of us had to follow the protocol of social distancing six feet apart. I was called in, and before entering the procedure room, my vitals were taken, including my weight, height, and blood pressure. The nurse explained the procedures that were to take place and assured me that Dr. Bird was super quick, so the appointment shouldn't be very long. I was relieved because my bladder was about to explode. I was told they would rather have me practically bursting with a full bladder. So, I refrained from running out of the room even though it took the doctor at least fifteen grueling minutes to see me.

"Hi Juliet, it's finally nice to meet you in person," Dr. Bird said.

"Yes, you too. I need to pee really badly," I said.

"That is fabulous! It's the best news I have heard all day."

"I am glad that this is good news for you."

"If you can hold off for about 5 minutes, that would be really helpful. When the bladder is full, it pushes down on the uterus and creates a straight path up for viewing."

"Okay, if it will help everything go smoothly, I think I can wait."

I was literally dying and about to burst. The other thing was that I got UTIs easily, thus I hated holding my bladder in general. When the ultrasound wand was inserted in, I felt tons of pressure on my bladder and was trying not to fidget from the discomfort. Dr. Bird navigated the wand toward my right ovary, counted three antral follicles, and measured them. Then, over to the left side, where there were four antral follicles, she measured them and exclaimed that she had found a few more than anticipated due to my AMH levels. So I had seven antral follicles, resting bodies that could turn into mature ones carrying viable eggs when stimulated with hormone injections. My suppression check seemed satisfactory, and we quickly moved on to the hysteroscopy.

My bladder was again greatly irritated by the speculum insertion. Dr. Bird sprayed a bit of lidocaine on my cervix so that while inserting the scope, it would be more comfortable. Once it was in, I stared at the screen to see the inside of my uterus and the fallopian tube openings. The endoscopic camera caused discomfort, and the nurse told me to wiggle my toes. All was looking good—my uterus had an extra straight canal because my bladder was pushing so hard on it. It was all swift. I asked questions about my antral follicles, but was so distracted by the discomfort in my abdomen and screen that I didn't understand what was being said. I thought it was possible to have more follicles grow with the hormone stimulation injections that had to start on Monday, but what was seen on the screen was what I had to work with. Thus, the goal was to have all seven follicles produce viable eggs.

That evening, Micah had to take four antibiotic pills to flush out his urethra of any bad bacteria. However, we knew antibiotics eliminated all bacteria, thus probiotic replenishment was definitely in the plan.

Did You Just Squirt Out $100?

On Monday evening, we started the hormone injections. When it came to IVF, all I thought about was the hormones my body needed to absorb. I was okay with needle pokes and had no phobias there. We had watched the videos the night before to prepare ourselves. During the injections, we had the video going as well to make sure we didn't mess up and inject me with incorrect doses of hormone. I was prescribed a daily dose of 450 IU, which was a very high dose of hormone and quite pricey. Micah tried to ensure no bubbles were in the syringe but then his rugged muscles accidentally squirted out about 75 IU!

"Did you just waste like a hundred dollars of hormone?" I asked.

"Um, I tried not to," Micah said.

"Oh my god, you have to be more careful because these hormones are not cheap!"

Apart from the mishap, Micah did super well with the Gonal injection, which didn't hurt. Next up was Menopur; for some reason, we didn't know how much had to be taken into the syringe. It was a different measuring unit, and we freaked out about how much 75 IU was for that needle. The whole vial was 75 IU, so we figured the entire dose was to be given. We would have known that if we had just watched the next thirty seconds of the video. My advice is to watch the videos on YouTube and not freak out. I also thought having my partner do the injections made him feel like he was part of the whole process. If you don't have a partner, you are fine doing the injections yourself. You can also get a friend to help out.

By day three of the stimulation injections, I wasn't feeling well. I watched one lady's vlog, and she mentioned being nauseous, so I waited for that to occur. I also did the castor oil packs every night to get blood flow in my abdomen. It felt like it helped me conceive the last two times I got pregnant, so why not? I couldn't move or do anything during these one-hour sessions, so I caught up with the previous two seasons of *Keeping Up With the Kardashians*. They produced nine children between all the sisters, so maybe I could visually imbibe their fertility.

An ultrasound was scheduled on Saturday to see if my follicles were progressing correctly. Let's go, ovaries! Let's go! Truly, I had no idea how my body would react to the hormones. I was excited but also anxious to see the results. During this first week, I felt so distracted by IVF and the pandemic. It wasn't easy to concentrate on anything else.

I had an important virtual round table coming up, which I was co-facilitating. My manager was attending, and that evening, she told my colleague and me that our director would also be on the call. I tried not to freak out and thought I was prepared enough. During my part of the presentation, I felt I could not answer a couple of questions; I had to call on my manager to get her input. I should have known this information, but I did not refresh myself on the data. Thus, I felt I was fumbling quite a bit. I was pretty embarrassed because it was in front of my director, and I was not as prepared as I should have been. Being a career woman and wanting to be a mommy simultaneously was tough. Yes, we women can multitask like bosses, but I think I was so distracted that I didn't know this group of health care practitioners would ask difficult questions about the presented data. I felt pretty disappointed in myself for not being on top of everything, but I realized that something had to give. When starting a family and having a career, the career usually suffers to some extent. This inevitable, unfair outcome was why I put having kids off until now. I had too many extra endeavours and items to accomplish. One of my older colleagues said she felt similarly before she had her son and realized that she never truly started living until after she had him. I felt that was a bit extreme, but what did I know?

Trying to conceive via IVF during a pandemic was stressful because getting ill anytime during my planned-out schedule would eff things up really well. We were being as vigilant as we could during these unprecedented times. By the way, if I hear the word unprecedented one more time, I will lose it. Its overuse during the pandemic was excruciating.

I had been ruminating about whether I would post my kids on my social media once they entered this world. Will they be trophies I can show off to the world? I went back and forth on this issue because I wanted my audience to applaud me for my intellect, creativity, and other amazing talents. I didn't want hundreds of likes because of my biology and ability to produce a child. Not that that shouldn't be recognized and celebrated, but I felt like I was much more than my ovaries. Plus, getting to this point was quite difficult and stressful. I didn't mind speaking about my journey because other women could hopefully learn from my experiences and not feel alone. My social media was quite public because of all my endeavours, but maybe after birth, it might be a good idea to be more private. Or, perhaps I wanted to make another social media account and turn my cute Shiba Inus and baby into significant influencers. I did spend a lot of money to obtain all of them. Why not make my money back, ya? God, I am such a Gemini.

15. Who Are You? And Where's My Doc?

I was excited yet slightly anxious about my first ultrasound after five days of stimulation injections. What if my body didn't react to the ridiculously high dose of hormones, which cost an excessive amount of money, mind you? I was diligently injecting the hormones into my tummy every evening. No pain, no gain. God, I sound like an 80s gym ad.

A strange male and a female assistant escorted me to the exam room at the doctor's office. Micah could not enter the examination room with me due to COVID restrictions. I was astonished that it wasn't my female doc doing my ultrasound. I had never had a male practitioner except when I was a child. He spoke about the plan for the day without introducing himself. I may have nodded or replied audibly; I was still shocked and wondered whether I was genuinely okay with this. Nobody informed me there would be different people doing my ultrasounds, and I suppose I had to understand that the schedule was not rigid with the pandemic. I also didn't want to be opposed to fair and equal opportunities for male practitioners to stick a wand up my vagina, either. Why couldn't a man do it professionally if a woman could do it professionally? So I tried to play it real cool, and truly, this man (who I found out later was one of the fertility docs) was highly professional and skillful. When he lifted the covering across my lap, it was barely enough so that he could quickly insert the wand and immediately cover me back up.

We viewed the left side of my ovaries, which had one follicle developing. The right side had three, two of which were a bit bigger. The mystery male doc finished measuring, pulled the wand out, and instructed me to sit back up.

"So it looks like you have four developing follicles; two of them seem to be growing more than the other two," the doctor said. "We will measure the follicles at the next appointment, and if they aren't progressing enough, we may need to stop this cycle and start again. We want an adequate number of mature follicles for egg retrieval, giving us the best chances to form a good number of embryos."

"Okay, what do you think my chances are of stopping this cycle?" I asked.

"I would say seventy-thirty. I think you will most likely go through egg retrieval. You already have your appointment scheduled for Tuesday, right?"

"Yes."

"Great, well, good luck."

"Thanks."

Directly after, I had to take a blood test, which was something that was done with every ultrasound. I wasn't quite sure what they were testing for, but I later learned that they wanted to keep track of my estrogen levels. I dreaded the possibility of halting this cycle if I wasn't responding correctly. Why would I let that go to waste if I had one quality egg? Was IUI a possibility if I wasn't heading towards an egg retrieval?

IVF Day Nine

I went in for my Tuesday ultrasound, and surprise, surprise, I had the same male doc once again who measured my four developing follicles. They all seemed to be growing, and the doc told me that Dr. Bird would ultimately decide on the next steps.

I finally received a call from my nurse, who told me to come back on Thursday and to continue taking my injections. I only had one more dose of the antagonist (Cetrotide), which I had to start Saturday evening. Essentially, this injection was halting ovulation so that the eggs could stay put and grow. My nurse advised me to call the pharmacy for the extra dose. I asked her if an IUI was possible if the doc decided to stop the cycle. She double-checked and confirmed that it was a possibility. I felt slightly relieved that all of these injections would not be entirely wasted, even if my chances of conception were decreased with IUI compared to IVF. This process was truly mentally exhausting.

IVF Day Eleven

I continued my castor oil packs along with two more days of injections. Come on, follicles, grow! Again, I was excited and anxious. To retrieve or not to retrieve? That was the ultimate question at my age. I was back at SRM and waited for the doc to enter the room. To my surprise, it was a woman. Yay!

"Hi, I'm Stephanie, and I will be your sonographer today. You have the same birthday as my daughter! Oh, Geminis!"

"Oh ya, I know Geminis, all right," I said.

"Yes, they just have a mind of their own and like to do things their way. My daughter can be somewhat stubborn," Stephanie said.

"We are quite independent."

"Yes, you guys are. My daughter has been living in San Francisco for a while and is now returning to Seattle. Guess it just wasn't for her."

"Mmm, I see."

"Okay, I am about to insert the wand, so you will feel some of the cold gel. Look at that uterus!"

"Ya, I was going to say the same thing," the assistant chimed in. "It looks like it should be in a textbook."

"Cool," I chided, flattered that my uterus should be THE example. I mean, how many women can say that about their reproductive parts (totally kidding btw)?

Stephanie read off a bunch of measurements and told me the doctor would have to take a look and decide from there. I went home and waited for my phone call.

Dr. Bird called a few hours after my appointment and indicated that I had nine follicles, four of which actually developed. I guess it depended on what the sonographer saw, and since I had multiple, maybe some were miscounted due to the 2D nature of the ultrasound. Two dominant larger ones on the right side were 22mm and 18mm. I had a third on the right that was 13.5mm and one on the left that was 13mm. Thus, the two were lagging a bit behind. Ideally, they liked to see three or more follicles of at least 15mm for egg retrieval.

"Ya, this cycle, unfortunately, doesn't seem as stellar as we had hoped," Dr. Bird said.

"Oh, okay." I was losing hope for the egg retrieval to occur.

"Your estrogen levels have increased to 1,154, which is good. So I would suggest that we have you take one more day of injections and hope the other two will perk up a bit."

"Okay, that sounds like a good plan."

"Yes, I think this is the best option, and I would do it as well."

Dr. Bird's personalizing this decision was comforting and gave me confidence.

"So, I do not want to waste the developed eggs. Thus, can we do an IUI if we halt the cycle?" I asked.

"Right, we can convert this to a medically treated IUI if we don't see any progression with the follicles. I will have the nurse call you very shortly so you can come by and pick up another day of medication."

I was a bit more on edge and was willing and begging my follicles to develop just a bit more. I did not tell any of my girlfriends that I started IVF, and right about now, it may have been an excellent time to get some support. However, I was just too exhausted after the two

61

miscarriages to speak about more pregnancy stuff again. In general, I was fine carrying this on my own, and maybe I just needed to keep it to myself for a little bit. Sometimes, when I speak about nerve-wracking things, I become more anxious. So, I kept mum about trying to be a mum again.

To Retrieve or Not to Retrieve.

It was IVF day twelve, and my tummy was now officially a dartboard with over twenty punctures. So far, the hormones have been manageable. I had a few bouts of crankiness and slight nausea, but staying hydrated and healthy helped.

During my castor oil pack hour, I had been *Keeping Up With the Kardashians*—literally. When I was on work travel, I watched them on TV because I was bored. It was quite entertaining to see what the K sisters were up to! There was one ridiculous episode where they ended the show with a food fight at Khloe's house to torment her OCD behaviors. The food waste was abhorrent and reeked of the rich and privileged. I almost wanted to stop watching the show right then; however, for some stupid reason, the show kept pulling me in. There was an episode I connected with when Khloe was contemplating having her eggs retrieved.

"Having your eggs retrieved is the best insurance policy you will ever have," Kourt said.

I was like, dude, you are speaking to the choir! I wish I could have done this when I was in my early thirties, but I was too busy obtaining a Master's and then a PhD. I had no money, although I probably should have used some of my student credit line or scholarships to fund this.

Khloe had about fifteen follicles, and they retrieved nine eggs, whereas five seemed to be of the highest quality. However, she debated on whether she should have another batch of her eggs fertilized with her partner's sperm just in case, and to be sure that she had some quality embryos. Because, truly, you are never quite certain how good your eggs are until fertilized and the initial stages of growth occur. I was impressed by her family planning and wished I had that knowledge before I turned thirty-five.

It was decision day. I prayed to all fertility goddesses to please cast growing spells on all four of my follicles, especially those lagging in growth. My sonographer that day was Julie, the name I was called growing up. The name Juliet came along when I worked retail in my early twenties at The Gap and Club Monaco, and when there was another Julie in my dental hygiene class. The coincidences during my ultrasound appointments continued at an entertaining rate. Maybe she even had the same birthday as me. Julie popped the wand inside me and wielded it around to view my ovaries. She measured, and I took mental notes. Every follicle grew a bit more, but the left was still slightly lagging at 14mm. The one on the right that was the smallest jumped from 13.5mm to 16mm! I was ecstatic; however, I wondered if this was good enough for Dr. Bird. I asked Julie whether or not she thought I would head toward an egg retrieval, and she said she was going to leave it up to the doc to make those decisions. I then asked about women who had to halt a cycle and restart. She mentioned that she had seen some improvements in these cases, but many have remained the same regarding the number of viable and mature follicles. My gut feeling, no pun intended, was that I had a solid number of follicles for egg retrieval. After my appointment, I told Micah that I knew these eggs were the ones and that, hopefully, Dr. Bird would think the same.

I waited a grueling bunch of hours, again distracted and antsy. Finally, I received a call from Dr. Bird. I was dying to hear what she thought of the progress. She reviewed the new measurements and was so happy to see that the follicles grew more; thus, we would schedule an egg retrieval. Omgahhhh! I was relieved as I wasn't sure if she thought the progression was good enough. I wonder if those castor oil packs did the trick by increasing the circulation in my abdomen. I was instructed to give myself an HCG trigger shot that evening at precisely nine as the egg retrieval was extremely time-sensitive. I was also instructed to take a pregnancy test to make sure the HCG levels in my system increased appropriately. On the day of my egg retrieval, which was scheduled thirty-six hours from my trigger shot, Micah would be coming in with me to do a sperm collection. They would tell me the number of eggs to be retrieved that day! This was all very exciting, and I hoped I would have a successful collection of viable eggs.

16. The Beauty of a Blackout

I was to have no food or water after midnight the evening before my egg retrieval. Saying you can't have water was like saying you couldn't breathe oxygen. OMG, I was going to die if I didn't have some water in the middle of the night after I woke up to take a pee. What if I dehydrated like a raisin? How would I prevent a possible surprise UTI? Seriously, the thought of being unable to drink water freaked me out. I would survive, I told myself.

In the morning, I had to remember not to have any water. It was such a habit. We were in the waiting room, and a nurse with many cool tattoos on her said she would take me back. I made Micah kiss me mask-to-mask; he was reluctant because everyone watched us. The nurse commented on how her boyfriend would never do that. I thought of something bratty in my head, like, well, then your boyfriend kinda sucks. I mean, if you're about to go under so that they can stick an enormous needle through your vaginal wall up into your ovaries and then vacuum your eggs out of your body, I think you deserve a bloody kiss, ya? Pandemic mask to pandemic mask.

The surgery center was a hospital ward with curtains and beds. I was surprised at the whole setting. For some reason, I thought it would just be more like an exam room, but I was going through surgery, so it made sense that everything should be hospital-grade. After changing into my gown, socks, and cap, my nurse returned to give me two extra-strength Tylenols and the tiniest cup of water.

"Live it up and drink it all!"

"Cheers."

And down they went. I was afraid I would need more water because sometimes the pills get stuck in my throat. But thank goodness they went down like melted butter.

My nurse went over things I may feel post-surgery and said I would be prescribed oxycodone if the pain was really bad. I looked at the prescription, and it was for one tablet. I knew I would not need it and was wondering if it was truly necessary to prescribe it in the first place to patients, especially with all of the addiction issues tied to the drug.

The fertility doc who was going to retrieve my eggs came in to introduce herself. I asked her how long she had been doing this, and she said she was one of the founders. Thank god, I thought, an egg retrieval master! Excellent. At that moment, I remembered a conversation I had with an OBGYN I met via my day job. She mentioned that the University of Washington OBGYN school almost went into shambles after the founders of SRM left the school to begin their lucrative business. I mean, could you blame them? They were helping people have babies and making a lot of money! So I asked my egg retrieval doc if she knew this particular OBGYN, obviously not mentioning the comment she made, and the fertility doc said that they go to the same church. Well, hail Mary Jesus, what a coincidence!

After that short convo, the anesthesiologist came in and went through his spiel, letting me know I would be conked out real good.

My nurse came in and told me to pee before we went into the operating room. I was already hooked up to the IV. She did a fabulous job, and I didn't feel anything. Cold stickers were placed on me as soon as I lay on the surgery bed. I asked why they were cold. It was as if they stuck them in the fridge, but it was just my body heat contrasting to the lucrative inanimate 3M inventions. The oxygen mask around my face made me cough a bit when I tried to breathe in. Within seconds, I was out.

I woke up in a daze and noticed that I was in the recovery bed. I was still so sleepy. The nurse came in to check on me. She gave me a juice box and some graham crackers.

"Did I say anything while I was out?" I asked.

"You spoke about watching Instagram stories, but obviously, that's not what you were doing."

Hmm, how funny that was. In my delirious state, all I talked about was social media. I sipped my juice box and gobbled my nommy crackers. I looked at the board on the wall to see what they wrote, which would indicate how many eggs were retrieved, and it said four! I was elated that I had four whole eggs they obtained from my ovaries! I was so scared that there would be none. The fertility doc came in to talk to me about my retrieval. She mentioned that all four eggs were retrieved on the right side, and the follicle on the left side was empty. Wow, I thought, you never know what you're gonna get. I had a surprise Easter egg on the right! The other follicles must have hidden it during the ultrasound. My right ovary was working overtime this round.

I had a good ten-minute conversation with the nurse; one of the topics was whether women in their early thirties should have their eggs retrieved as insurance since, as we age, the quality and quantity of the eggs decrease exponentially. According to her experience, she had seen it all and didn't necessarily recommend it to everyone. She had seen women in their twenties who don't produce as many eggs compared to some women in their thirties. I was a bit astonished hearing this. In general, I do think it is better to be on the safe side and consider the quality of your fertility well before your mid-thirties.

I got dressed, and the nurse walked me to the main entrance of the building. I felt okay, and there was no pain yet. My nurse sent me home with a bunch of extra-strength Tylenol, and I knew I wouldn't have to use the prescription for one pill of oxycodone. I took the turquoise socks too because everyone said always to take your hospital socks. So I did as a souvenir.

I rested in bed and slept for most of the day. I had some dull abdomen pain later in the afternoon. I took a Tylenol at 4:30 pm and then another before bedtime. The next day, I felt totally fine. I was completely impressed with the entire procedure. I was seriously expecting the worst in terms of pain and was proven wrong. We prayed to ourselves and to whoever was listening in the various galaxies of the universe that all was going okay with the embryos and that all four would develop properly. Grow, babies, grow!

17. Anticipation Volume One Million

I received a call mid-afternoon the next day from one of the nurses. She first said, "We have scheduled your embryo transfer."

OMG! One or some of my embryos made it! I wanted to know right away how many made it.

"That will be the second part of the conversation," the nurse said.

So, after a few minutes of discussing the day of the embryo transfer, which was in two days, I was told I had two embryos that had developed. I was slightly sad that all four didn't grow, but beggars couldn't be choosers, ya? I was grateful for what had transpired. I still had viable eggs, but this was only another step up the very tall ladder.

<u>Let's Get These Babies Transferred</u>

It was the morning of my embryo transfer. I was nervous and excited, which seemed to be the default feeling of this whole process. I again had to come in with a full bladder, just like my very first appointment for the hysteroscopy and mock run-through. I was led to a dim room with a curtain to block the door I just entered. I was wearing a dress, so all I had to do was take off my underwear, which was much more convenient than taking my pants off. I sat in the cushy, white lounge-like chair and noticed a sliding door opposite where I entered. I assumed the lab was back there because people were chatting and laughing. I had to pee so bad I swore my bladder would burst at any moment. The instructions were to consume a liter of water, and I knew I would never be able to hold that much water in my bladder for the next hour. Big tip of the day: You know your body best. The sonographer finally came in, and it was the same one who had the daughter with the same birthday as me. She put some warm gel on the ultrasound wand, and this time it went on my tummy, not in my vagina, which was atypical compared to my past appointments.

"So your bladder is full, so I want you to empty some urine. I don't want you to be too uncomfortable for the transfer."

"Really? Well, how much should I empty?" I was in shock yet relieved that I could expel some pee.

She grabbed a coffee cup from the cupboard. "How about three-quarters worth in this cup? You can stop yourself midstream, and it will be easy. Your bladder will fill up again really quickly."

I thought about how I had once tried to stop myself midstream when I was giving a sample for a UTI, and it didn't work at all. I was doubtful that I could do it properly. I went next door to the washroom and didn't even bother putting my underwear back on. It felt amusing to pee in a coffee cup. I started peeing, and the cup filled up so fast that I thought I was not going to be able to stop for the life of me. I clenched my kegel muscle, and remarkably, I could control my flow. Hallelujah! I poured the coffee cup of pee into the toilet and threw the cup in the trash. I returned to the room as quickly as possible and waited ten minutes before Dr. Bird and the sonographer entered.

The embryologist opened the sliding door and exclaimed, "Your embryos are very good-looking."

That proclamation was the best symphony that has ever entered my ears.

Dr. Bird mentioned their happiness with these results and gave me a photo of my two little circles. These balls of replicated cells were quite cute. One embryo was slightly ahead in development compared to the other one and was already in the morula stage. The one slightly lagging was in the 8-cell stage. I stared at the photo, bewildered at the myriad of activities involved in arriving at this place. Even though I was not pregnant yet, I still felt a great sense of accomplishment and relief. Our bodies could produce a zygote; it just needed extra external assistance.

Before we did the actual transfer, Dr. Bird did a mock run where the empty catheter was placed into my uterus. This was to ensure everything was properly visible on the screen and the path was clear. It was quite interesting to watch the whole process via the ultrasound. I was able to see the catheter being pushed through and then out. I had no discomfort as a numbing agent was sprayed on my cervix prior to insertion.

The screen switched to the lab, and I could see my two cute embryos. Dr. Bird read my patient number three times to ensure these were actually my embryos being transferred (I wondered how often that mistake occurred). The embryologist confirmed and got the catheter ready to load up the microscopic babies. Once they were sucked up from the petri dish, the screen switched back to my ultrasound. The embryologist handed Dr. Bird the loaded catheter, and we were ready for transfer. Dr. Bird spoke through each step, and I watched as the catheter went into my uterus.

She released them to complete the transfer. We waited a few moments while the catheter was still inserted. The embryos were way too tiny to show up on the ultrasound, so I just had to imagine them being squirted into my body. I didn't feel a thing except that I had to pee again. Doc said I had about a twenty to twenty-five percent chance of having twins. I had an appointment in ten days to do a blood test and check if HCG was at all detected. In general, I was quite impressed with the whole transfer process. It was efficient, and everything went smoothly. This entire team was made up of highly skilled professionals, and I was grateful to them.

Am I Pregnant?

It had been a week and a half since my transfer. There was some anxiousness, but I felt okay overall. Tomorrow would be my blood test appointment. I had some chest tenderness earlier in the week and felt tired. Because I couldn't wait for the blood test results, I took two pregnancy tests. Both were positive. I knew they would be because of my early pregnancy symptoms, which I was pretty familiar with now thrice over.

The pandemic precautions were still in place, and apparently, Seattle may open up at the end of May, which would be in a phased approach, with each lasting about three weeks. The county continued to monitor cases to determine whether they needed to go back a phase or forge forward.

Everyone in Seattle was over it, and many ignored the precautions. However, some adhered quite strictly and wore masks at all times in public. It was definitely more enforced at the grocery stores, and I felt there was obedience in our community. Some of the Americans were funny; they protested over the dumbest things. When the government was trying to protect them, they felt their rights were being violated, so they screamed bloody murder, marched together in large groups with no masks because it was a free country, and therefore could do whatever they wanted. The result was a surge in COVID-19 cases. Smdh. In Asian countries, there is more of a group mentality where if one fails, we all fail, so they act in harmony. I wish Americans possessed more of this behavior and realized that it's not just about them but a collective, which consists of frail individuals who cannot fight off disease like healthy people.

Happy Mummy's Day!!

I went to the clinic on Mother's Day for my blood test. I hoped my home pregnancy tests and symptoms were accurate. I received a call that same day, and my HCG levels were at 297.5! I was preggy! A value of fifty or greater was normal. I had to make another appointment in three days to make sure the HCG levels were increasing appropriately.

Wednesday's Blood Test

The nurse called me on Wednesday afternoon while we were walking the pups. My HCG levels quadrupled compared to the first blood draw! They increased to 1240! What a relief. My TSH levels were normal, thank goodness. I had to make an ultrasound appointment in three weeks. Dr. Bird said I had a 70% chance of live birth at this moment. After the first ultrasound, there would be a 90% success rate. Micah mentioned he always held his breath when listening to the phone calls.

During the next few weeks, I became more bloated, developed some pimples, and felt more tired. I finally had the courage to cut my bangs, which turned out pretty well. When COVID restrictions became more lax, I no longer needed to see the hairdresser every few weeks like before. I also began googling the foods I ate to make sure I was not poisoning the baby. It seemed the stress shifted from one topic to the next during this journey.

Meanwhile… Through this pandemic, unrest unfolded as radically patriotic Americans protested against public pandemic measures, i.e., stay-at-home, business closures, mask-wearing, etc. These folks gathered in large crowds at legislative buildings, not socially distancing or wearing masks. Even the anti-vaxxers come out of their caves to spew non-factual data and proclaim how they would not be forced to get a COVID-19 vaccine. Even if there was a vaccine that worked, not everyone had access to the vaccine. The first shipment was to go to frontline healthcare workers and high-risk patients. The dissemination of misinformation in the media was exhausting to watch. By the first of June, Seattle was still not ready to open up.

More importantly, America was in turmoil not just from the pandemic but from the systemic racism that had been buried in the foundation of this land from day one, which contaminated many people like an airborne virus. A series of extremely violent and racist video-recorded events occurred to Black people since the beginning of the pandemic that has created a burning fury across the nation. These events were the last dominos to be placed, which sent the whole row tumbling into chaos.

Ahmaud Arbery was jogging in the park when he was hunted down by white males and shot in broad daylight while an accomplice video-recorded the murder.

George Floyd was sent to death by a Caucasian officer with unreasonable brute force. The cop suffocated George as he pushed his knee on George's neck, all the while acting like he was bragging about his prized trophy. George cried out that he couldn't breathe and then stopped breathing.

Christian Cooper was bird-watching in Central Park when he told a white lady to leash her dog. This "Karen" was astonished that her white privilege and self-entitlement were being threatened and questioned, so she weaponized the color of her skin. She called the cops and lied about her safety, which could have endangered Christian and potentially send him to death like George Floyd. Luckily, Christian recorded the whole charade. This *Karen* was fired from her job, and her dog was taken away.

71

There had been three days of riots across the nation. Peaceful protests were not showcased on the news; only acts of violence from rioters, anarchists, and cops. Building windows were smashed, cars were set on fire, and people were shot at with rubber bullets or pepper-sprayed. This pandemic was truly unprecedented (I still can't stand to hear that word and need a thesaurus). This was the first time I saw a full-blown outcry, maybe even a revolution, from the public. Yet, many remained silent. Some of my Black friends, via social media, called out their white friends for their lack of support and notified them that they were watching closely. The white fragility I encountered was astonishing. Many non-BIPOCs did not understand the systemic racism and oppression in America and, unfortunately, chose not to become more informed. This is still the case today.

The privilege and entitlement continued the vicious racist cycle. The thought of people not being woke due to choice hit a little harder because I was going to be bringing a child into this world. This was the state of the society at the moment—one where I was constantly outraged for many reasons. The presidential choices were two old white men who were sexual predators and imbeciles. It was energy-draining and depressing, and I acknowledged my privilege of even saying this within the safety of my home.

First Ultrasound Since Transfer

I had been so distracted, livid, and frustrated with what I encountered during the Black Lives Matter (BLM) protests. The violence and brutality of police against peaceful protesters was excruciating. Defunding and dismantling the police force was mandatory now. Seattle even had a few nights' curfew from all the riots downtown. Ultimately, the police stood down, the precinct in Capitol Hill was boarded up, and the protesters began their occupation in the area. Initially, they labeled it CHAZ (Capitol Hill Autonomous Zone), but then folks felt that it was taking away from the actual movement. So then it was called CHOP (Capitol Hill Organized Protest), but on social media, many referred to it as CHOP/CHAZ for those unfamiliar with the modification. What was also a considerable distraction was trying to educate some Asian friends of mine who seriously did not get it at all. They commented how not all cops were bad apples (obviously) or asked, "Did you know George Floyd was a criminal?" All of which did nothing for BLM or the oppression and racism Black people faced for the last 400 years in America. I fought hard, typing like a mad Kermit the Frog, but it was futile. Those people were so blinded by their privilege and being a "model minority."

Anyhow, I arrived for my ultrasound, and as soon as I took off my underwear and covered myself with the sheet, I started a video chat with Micah so he could be part of the appointment. Dr. Bird came in pretty quickly, and we got right to it. I looked at the screen and tried to make sure Micah could see, too, but the screen was on the wall, so it was a bit far for the chat. I saw the little baby, and it was so cute. Dr. Bird started measuring various things and pointed out the heartbeat was beating at a healthy rate. It looked like a really quick fluttering right under the baby's small head. Micah unfortunately couldn't see it due to the quality of the chat. The assistant started snapping screenshots. Dr. Bird said I was seven and a half weeks along, and the due date would be January 17, 2021, a week before Micah's birthday! I was in such a daze that everything felt surreal, and I couldn't pay proper attention to anything happening. Also, the video chat was distracting. Stupid pandemic! I was happy, though, because everything looked healthy. Things were progressing. I was told to make an appointment with my OBGYN in the next few weeks.

During the sixth and seventh week, the potential to feel nauseous significantly increased. I was adamant about not getting too hungry, which would make the nausea come quickly. Thus, every time I was hungry, I ate right away. Avoiding ralphing was the name of the game. It was exhausting figuring out what to eat every couple of hours. I was so tired from eating so often. There were times when I was just too tired but also hungry, so I felt like cry-eating because I just wanted to go to sleep. It was pitiful, which I gathered from Micah's reactions. Soda pop was my bestie. I loved the lavender dry soda, ginger beer, and plain carbonated water, which all helped the heartburn or indigestion feeling. I also wanted cold drinks, which was bizarre. My appetite for yogurt and fruit skyrocketed, and I couldn't get enough. I sent Micah to the store multiple times during the day to get me watermelon, cherries, and white peaches. Because I had to eat so often, I tried to purchase food that was easy to prepare or had no prep time. My easy go-tos were bagels and cream cheese, blocks of cheese, crackers, nuts, veggies and dip, and bananas.

I felt a little sorry for Micah, too, because once the stimulation injections began during the IVF cycle, we had not had sex in two months. When I knew I was pregnant, I did not want to risk uterine contractions at all. There was no conclusive research that sex was harmful, but if I wanted to decrease uterine contractions, I believed that I should abstain until I was close to the end of the first trimester. This was something we discussed with Dr. Bird as well, who mentioned that not having sex at all during the pregnancy was crazy. (I wasn't going to do that to Micah or me.) She did advise that waiting until my ten-week mark would probably be safer, which would fall on Father's Day. Lucky Micah!

Lately, I have been trying not to stress myself out with all the craziness in the world and refraining from getting involved in social media fights, which generally was never worth it. I was still tired often and usually took a midday nap. I also hadn't told some of my close girlfriends because I was scared. The PTSD from the previous pregnancies was real. I planned to share my good news with friends at the second-trimester mark. This time, I was trying hard to keep it a secret, which was a little silly, perhaps, but I didn't want to jinx myself a third time.

I participated in a COVID-19 pregnancy study called ASPIRE. The study required me to indicate each day if I had certain symptoms and was supposed to take blood samples. The kits, unfortunately, were delayed.

I wanted to do more art, but some of the media was toxic. Even Micah didn't want me painting due to the risks to the fetus. Sigh.

I also just had my COVID birthday with a beautiful COVID cake. I had to work during the day, so we didn't do much. In the evening, we ordered some takeout sushi from our usual go-to spot, and they always gave us a special treat for free because they liked us so much. They were the sweetest. We ended up at Volunteer Park in the big field with the brick theatre stage. It was lovely; the weather was nice, and we felt relaxed. Cheers to thirty-nine!

Ultrasound #2

I again had to arrive alone for my second ultrasound with the continued COVID restrictions. My appointments from now on were to be at my

OBGYN office. At this first appointment, I was being seen by the physician assistant (PA) I saw during my second miscarriage. I remembered her name. Every time I stepped into the OBGYN office, my PTSD was triggered as it was always bad news with them. I needed to be less superstitious, but sometimes I wanted to change the office because I felt it was bad luck to go back. However, I didn't and hoped that things would be much different this time—that it would be more successful and joyous.

After I had my blood pressure checked by one of the techs, I had to remove all of my clothes and put a "robe" on—it was basically a paper bag. I also gave Micah a ring on FB video chat so he could be part of the events. The PA came in and reminded me that she had seen me before. I told her I remembered her. We started with some questions and then the ultrasound. She popped the wand in me, and I saw something, but I hoped it looked normal. Their portable machine was so old that the resolution was inferior, and it was a dinosaur compared to what SRM had. She pointed out the heartbeat, and I saw a slight flickering. She took a measurement and said I was nine weeks and six days along. It was a speedy viewing that I didn't get to savor for as long as I wished I could.

I received a printout of a blob—my 2D baby. The rest of the appointment consisted of a breast check, a cervical swab for chlamydia and gonorrhea, and explanations of what to expect next. I was told I would be receiving a call from the testing clinic, which would take my blood and check for genetic disorders and abnormal chromosomal activity. An ultrasound was to be done as well. My next appointment was in a month with my actual OBGYN doc, and every month after that, I was to come in and have my baby's heartbeat checked with the Doppler machine. I received blood work that day as well and went to the third floor only to wait for an hour and have five test tubes of blood collected. It was a waste of time, and Micah asked me if it was necessary since SRM had all my recent blood work. I didn't even realize to ask at the time. He was also wondering why they didn't measure the heartbeat. I thought it was because the machines sucked and didn't have the capabilities.

18. It's Been Awhile

It has been about three months since Micah and I had sex. The past two miscarriages left me in a state, and the thought of having sex within the first trimester freaked me the eff out. Micah was probably dying a little but knew it was all worth it. He even thanked me for having to go through all of the IVF and pregnancy stuff. Well, I was almost eleven weeks along when we had sex. I was more tense and told him to go slow. After a minute or so, I wanted him to ensure there wasn't any bleeding. We were clear. Probably not the most romantic, but he was happy and satisfied.

"Was it like the first time?" I asked, eyes wide.

"Almost!" He said with a big, goofy grin.

I was relieved there was no bleeding and hoped to keep it that way. Afterward, we went downstairs to watch *Arrested Development* and *Jeopardy*. My *Jeopardy* skills were sharper than Micah's. (I am only just a bit competitive.) Maybe this was making the baby smarter!

So my tummy was getting bigger, and I was showing, which seemed early, but my girlfriend said it was because I was petite. My boobs and body felt extra itchy. I usually used this prescribed cream for my rashes, but I refrained because I didn't want my body to absorb extra chemicals that could be harmful. However, I would be at twelve weeks next week, and supposedly, getting your hair dyed was okay. My roots were in dire need of a bleaching.

Did I mention I had been working from home since the pandemic? That had been a blessing for the IVF and the first trimester. Things at work were going quite well, and I was fortunate I still had my career. A month ago, news articles stated that over forty million people in the US filed for unemployment. That was horrifying to think about. Micah and I had been so fortunate that our companies still thrived during these tumultuous times. Mine was growing. Due to the threat of co-infection of the flu and COVID-19, influenza vaccines have been in very high demand lately. My role is within medical affairs, where I have a variety of responsibilities, the main ones being educating on the science and data, gathering insights from my territory, and collaborating with influenza experts. Micah is in natural supplements, and during the pandemic, customers, especially those who were against the vaccines, ran to the shelves to stock up on natural pills and remedies.

Nom Nom

I thought I had some super taste buds, but that has quadrupled since I became pregnant. Everything tasted incredibly delicious, most likely a primitive protective power pregnant ladies acquired to ensure they weren't eating poison. I had some fresh steamed corn on the cob with nothing on it, and it tasted like corn from the gods!

The smells of a particular food could turn my nose the other way. For example, Thai food and even some Vietnamese dishes from my own culture gave off too much potent odor for me to ingest. When Micah ordered them, I had to leave the room. Those organic peanut butter cracker bites became my best friends. The Ritz ones were a favorite back when I was a kid. Also, so were the whole wheat crackers (the organic Triscuit version) and cheese. Thank god it was cherry season because I ate many of those, along with white peaches. In general, more bland foods did better with me. I was approaching twelve weeks, and I still hadn't ralphed yet. Knock on wood.

That coming Thursday, I had an appointment for the nuchal translucency ultrasound and cell-free fetal DNA testing. We would also be learning the sex of the baby through these tests!

Upside Down Baby

We arrive at the Swedish Maternal & Fetal Specialty Center for our ultrasound and genetic counseling. I again was to come with a full bladder. I knew better about myself and allowed it to be about half full. Micah was able to go with me. I'm unsure why they had more lax protocols while still amid the pandemic, but I didn't question it. The first task was the ultrasound. The sonographer told me to get on the lounger, I asked if I should take my underwear off, as this was what I was accustomed to doing for ultrasound scanning. She said not yet as we would try to view the baby through my tummy. I was a bit embarrassed as to my readiness to take my undies off in front of strangers. I guess I just became so comfortable doing it.

One of the best things about this clinic was that we didn't have to take any photos or videos—they sent us a link to what the sonographer snapped and recorded after our appointment. Our baby was a funny little thing, upside down and horizontal. The wand was pushed into my tummy to turn the baby around slightly. We viewed all the limbs, the heartbeat, and its little mouth, which was moving. Being able to watch my baby move was magical. Its length was only about 2.5 inches long, but on screen, it looked huge. The nuchal translucency test was to check the fluid behind the baby's neck and measure it. Our baby's fluid was just over 1mm thick, which was considered normal. Anything more than 3mm could indicate Down syndrome or heart issues. After the sonographer had made her measurements, she said that she would write her report and that we would wait to see the genetic counselor. We were nervous and hoped her report would indicate that our baby was normal.

Our genetic counselor was Ursula. We followed her to her office with anxious excitement. She first mentioned that our baby's ultrasound results looked normal. What a relief! She explained that her job was to give us all of the options and information we needed to make informed decisions about what additional genetic tests we wanted to complete. I appreciated her candidness. At thirty-nine, the risk for chromosomal abnormality was less than two percent. If we took into consideration the normal ultrasound results, it decreased to one percent. Thus, the chances of our baby having an abnormal chromosome count were very small. This led us to the conversation of whether we wanted to do the cell-free DNA test where my blood would be drawn and tested for Down syndrome (trisomy 21), Edward's syndrome (trisomy 18), and Patau syndrome (trisomy 13). All of these cause developmental abnormalities. The other benefit of the test was that it deciphered the sex! From the discussion with the genetic expert, I had a feeling that my chances for those abnormalities would be quite low. Thus, it would mainly be to test for gender.

Ursula also allowed us to have the blood sample go to another lab not associated with the maternal center. Invitae Labs gave us the option of paying a $99 flat rate or going with our insurance, and they gave us an estimation of what our insurance may charge. I was kind of over all the blood draws and decided to opt out of the cell-free DNA test. If I wanted to change my mind, I could always come back for a blood draw. Since everything looked normal, my next ultrasound would be at twenty weeks, during which meticulously detailed measurements would be taken, showcasing any other developmental abnormalities. The sex would also be determined at this time. I thought maybe I could wait another two months to find out. After less than twenty-four hours of processing, we both did not want to wait that long.

I came back to the maternal center after the weekend and got my blood drawn. The results will be ready in a week or so! Oh, indecisive pregnancy brain.

19. Pandemic Pandemonium

The US was a bloody shizz show as the leadership and response to the COVID-19 pandemic had been moronic and irresponsible. Certain states (Texas, Florida, Arizona, California, and New York) opened up way too quickly and liberally from stay-at-home mandates. Restaurants, beaches, shops, hair/nail salons, basically all public spaces were up and ready to welcome guests and their money. I can't blame them; the economy tanked when the pandemic hit, and people needed to pay their bills and feed their families. However, the recklessness of mainly younger folks who wanted to party and have fun led to wildfire breakouts of COVID-19. Hospitals again were inundated with severely ill patients. By August 1st, 2020, the US had almost 4.7 million cases, which accounted for 26% of cases worldwide. The other issue was that some Americans were outraged about mask mandates, which they deemed unconstitutional. According to the 10th Amendment, states have the right to control the spread of disease within their jurisdiction. Thus, it was not unconstitutional. Incredibly, other nations and their citizens understand the necessity of being dutiful to ward off disease. Instead, in the land of the free, people genuinely didn't care about risking the safety and well-being of others. There was no acting as a collective in America. Instead, unintelligent people chose to utilize their liberties and hold COVID parties with the delusion they'd be able to overcome the illness without consequences. Unfortunately and unsurprisingly, I read about guests and even family members who came into contact with the partygoers who succumbed to their deaths after the festivities. The rhetoric that COVID was a hoax for many Americans was utterly baffling. It was evident how politically divided the country was, along with the gaps within the educational system. The amplification of non-factual, fear-mongering media was just too easy.

I tried to be a vigilant pregnant person. We wore masks in public as much as possible; it was always on at the grocery store. We saw a small number of friends outdoors and at a distance. I had to keep reminding Micah not to touch his face if he hadn't sanitized his hands. Pandemic practices and the BLM movement created huge divides, and social media was a burning inferno of animosity. One of my closest girlfriends posted an IG story about her being on a boat with a group of people close together to take the photo, and no one had their mask on. Recently, she had been quite opinionated about other folks who were not behaving safely, so I called her out about her hypocrisy. She told me I was wrong to think she wasn't being safe and that everyone on the boat got tested regularly. I retorted that trusting strangers was naive, and I didn't hear from her in the last few weeks. I could tell she was pissed at me because usually, she called me at least every other day or messaged me regularly. Was she insulted that I thought she was acting so careless? Perhaps. It seemed we got into a bit of a rift every summer and needed to take a little break from each other. It was astonishing to watch how the pandemic and the BLM movement divided people. Maybe there was too much virtue signaling and not enough benefit of the doubt.

The ongoing protests became increasingly hostile by the day. In Portland, federal agents were sent in with an onslaught of heightened brutality toward the protesters. Many were even arrested and placed in unmarked cars, which was technically kidnapping. Seattlelites continued their march and stood in solidarity with Portlanders to fight against police brutality (during protests) and for BLM. The Seattle Police Department (SPD) spared no one, not even the media, who were wearing proper ID badges. They were promised that this was how they would be differentiated from the protesters, but they were not immune to the assaults. During live streams, I watched journalists and their production team being shot at with flash bombs or rubber bullets and being maced/pepper sprayed directly in the face. The violence from SPD was horrific. Citizens have the right to protest, but they were not given the chance to do so.

20. M or F?

Well, enough of America the depressing. I suppose you are waiting in anticipation of our cell-free DNA test results. We were having a boy!!

One of the genetic counselors gave us a ring within a week of my blood draw and let us know that there was no indication of any trisomies. Our baby had a proper set of 23 chromosomes! So get this: both of us thought we would have a girl first, and the news of a boy gave us a bit of a shock! Micah asked if I was okay. LOL! I was happy that I even got to have a child. If it was healthy, that was all I wanted. Micah, for some reason, thought that he would only have daughters. I can't blame him since five girls and two boys are on his side, and then four nieces and one nephew. All in all, we were elated and still astonished! My tummy continued growing, and I could no longer hide my pregnancy.

It's Growing!!

I was seventeen weeks along, and my tummy was big. I measured my waist, and it was thirty-six inches. Micah beamed that we now had the same waist size. I still hadn't ralphed, which amazed me. My next ultrasound was in three weeks and would be a very detailed one. I had less heartburn, my boobs were still sore, and my nipples were darker. There were some headaches, neck pain, and aching joints and hips. I napped daily. Walking uphill left me out of breath; being pregnant was fun (insert sarcasm). The pregnancy brain was real, too! I felt a bit forgetful, and I was not as articulate. Or, maybe that was me getting older, too. Sigh. Recent evidence does showcase a decrease in grey matter for pregnant people, so it truly is a head-to-toe evolution! I felt some movement or fluttering from the baby at least once daily. I got a bit scared when it had been a while, and it seemed he wasn't moving. But then I'd feel a big boof and become so relieved.

COVID was still a prominent contagious figure worldwide, and Seattle was stuck in phase 2, which equated to some indoor dining and retail shopping being allowed. We wanted to head to Hawaii again in the fall, but it seemed too risky, although I heard the flights weren't full.

Something quite important to prevent during pregnancy was urinary tract infections (UTIs). It is so common and preventable, although I don't think many know what to do if they have recurring UTIs. For me, I figured out that putting kefir (I used Nancy's Organic Kefir, natural flavor, but any will do) on my urethra every night, even after I pee in the middle of the night, prevented UTIs for over a year! I put some on my finger and placed the kefir under my clitoris, where my urethra is. Taking antibiotics for UTIs is far too common and can lead to the development of resistance to the bacteria, potentially allowing superbugs to emerge and rendering the antibiotics ineffective. Additionally, what is needed is a replenishment of beneficial microflora in the area. Some women may also naturally harbor E. coli in their bladder. I think I am one of those. What didn't work was cranberry juice and D-Mannose pills/powder, which almost gave me diabetes. It's essentially a sugar that may help eliminate bacteria within the urinary tract. I made sure we were both clean before sex, and I tried to pee after sex, wiped myself, and placed kefir on my urethra. I also took oral probiotics along with Vitamin C daily. So far so good!

We announced our baby on social media around week eighteen and received plenty of congrats and support. I thought we were quite witty with our letter board, which stated "Gosh Dang-Cain Baby January 2021," for the photo with our cute little Shiba Inus. One of my SILs dryly commented that she hoped "Gosh" wasn't the baby's first name—eye roll. To offer some context, this SIL is usually sarcastic, but I sometimes felt that the vibes between us were a bit off. We also provided a poll for the gender reveal, and most guessed a girl. There were many comments about how some were waiting for our baby because they thought it would be gorgeous. Talk about pressure. Like, we aren't that good-looking of a couple, are we? Truly, I just hoped the baby would be healthy. If it were super cute, then that would be a double bonus! Why is society so vain? LMAO!

I feel like I have a sensitivity towards mothers who have gender disappointment. There have been way too many stories about how these moms have two of the same gender and then they have a surprise pregnancy for the third, and it's the same gender, or they have always wanted at least one boy and one girl, but can't come to terms with not having exactly what they wanted or planned for. Basically, it's a very controversial topic, yet I grow weary of the disappointment from these moms. I noticed that some women regretted aborting the surprise baby since it was a miracle. Others are pro-choice but would not be able to stand by the decision to terminate based on gender discrimination. Truthfully, I was appalled whenever I saw these posts online because I knew how difficult it was to conceive a child. Not only did I work extremely hard to prep my body, but the emotional toll IVF can have on an individual is not something to shrug off. Oh, and miscarrying twice didn't help either. I am very pro-choice, mind you. Thus, if this mother truly wanted to end this pregnancy, that was entirely her choice. What I found appalling was that people couldn't be happy with the gifts they were given. In this case, it was a healthy child. People can be so hung up on their perfect plans and high expectations. To me, that's kind of gross and sad at the same time. Life isn't about your exact plan being executed in fine detail; life is full of surprises. What we make of them and how we celebrate makes living worthwhile. If some mothers need to abort because they can't afford another child, that is entirely valid.

Gender preference is a hard argument. I read about how legacies wouldn't be continued if they didn't have a son, and there was pressure from all sides, including these mothers, to create a boy. Eff legacy! Why can't the daughters continue their legacy and keep their last names? In fact, why can't more men take their wives' last names? I was adamant about our child having both our last names. I think it's a good collaboration. Male legacy is so archaic, so patriarchal, and I am so over it. The posts indicating that gender disappointment was a real thing were something I couldn't comprehend. This was one thing I couldn't empathize with, and I found it difficult to even sympathize with, given my own circumstances.

Sunflower Fields Forever

We had a super busy day on Monday of my 20th week. Micah was trying to get my art supplies to the storage unit to make more room for baby stuff in the second bedroom (also my "office"). We also had our 20-week ultrasound early in the afternoon. It was quite a detailed session and took the whole hour. The sonographer had a list of the body parts, skeleton, and measurements she had to view. It made me a bit tired, especially since I was lying down, which was usually my nap time. Our baby was in an upside-down position, all curled up. There were some funny instances where he was doing a little dance with his feet and one shot showing us the palm of his hand. We even saw the male parts, so it was truly official. Micah and I half expected the sonographer to tell us it was a girl. We were still in disbelief it was a boy. We needed to have the baby face up, so the ultrasound wand was being jiggled on my tummy to make him move, which wasn't working, so then I was told to turn slightly to rest on my left side. Little baby didn't want to budge, so the lady went to write up her report while I continued to lay on my side, hoping he would move. After about 10-15 minutes, the radiologist told us everything looked normal, and the baby was 14 ounces and in the 85th percentile. He also wanted to look at the profile and the right arm, which was not viewable. Eventually, our baby moved himself, and we got a profile shot. We felt relieved that our baby was healthy. Another pregnancy milestone was met!

After this, we hurried to complete our storage errand, gobbled down a late lunch, and rushed home to get ready. I decided to head to the sunflower fields at the last minute since the sky was clear and sunny. I wore a white lacey maternity dress that my girlfriend handed down to me.

After purchasing our tickets, we hopped on a tractor to take a short ride across the highway and into the acres filled with sunflowers. We only had so much time before the sun set, and I planned to take some sweet maternity shots and do a gender reveal video. I purchased the deal where you can fill a large mason jar with flowers, and we set out on our hunt for the best-looking ones. It was a lot of fun seeking the most unique sunflowers; you felt like you were on a mission. We stopped a few times to take photos, and it was somewhat difficult with the sun's angle and the flowers' height. I highly suggest someone to assist you, like a professional photographer. Micah had to grab a small table for me to stand on, which was not very stable, and who knew how good my balance was with this baby bump? We found a sweet spot for some couples' pics, which took the longest because Micah wasn't happy with how his hair looked, so we did several takes, and he had to run back and forth to and from the camera as we didn't have a remote. With the blazing sun and exerted force, he got sweaty and hot, which didn't make for pretty pics - poor thing. I also tried not to get stung by the bumblebees that would feed off my cut flowers. We finally settled on a few that looked good enough and marched further to find a spot to do our virtual reveal video. We found a place with a barrel and wheel that was farm-style and perfect. It took only one take, and we were even in sync for one part of the video... the cherry on top. Truly, I had such a wonderful and giddy time in those fields. There was just magic in the air, and I was all smiles! Micah was such a good sport. Best IG husband ever!

My baby posts on social media received quite the attention. The congrats were appreciated; however, as I said before, I wished society would support women's endeavors not associated with their reproductive biology. Having a baby is a big deal, but I wish I had the same support for my art and other projects. I also had a distaste for all the blue hearts after posting the gender reveal. I mean, yes, it is a boy, but it doesn't mean we need to continue the outdated association of colors with gender. The other issue was comments about how Micah must be so excited because it was a boy. Like, because he is male, he should only want a boy? What is this, old-school China? The patriarchy is well and alive still, unfortunately, even in some of my friends, who I suppose are not as progressive as they should be or as I would expect them to be. Of course, I had to set the record straight and tell them that Micah wanted a girl and that we expected it to be a girl. They seemed a bit shocked because he was so rugged. Smdh. I have a penchant for being insulted somehow, even though people don't have that intent. Perhaps I expect too much from others in today's modern times. Levels of "wokeness" vary, and this was something I had to accept.

That week, we had to get our baby registry together. At first, I started with Target and learned about Baby List, which allowed you to add from anywhere on the web and even provide a button in your bookmarks to click and add quickly. Super convenient. We tried to keep it pretty basic yet cute. I was told zip-up one-piece body suits were convenient and to even add diapers and wipes even though it wasn't that fun of a present.

Since we had too many folks on the list, we decided to do two baby showers - one with my girlfriends and the other with Micah's family. My best girlfriend was so sweet to offer to organize and host the girls one on top her newly decorated rooftop. She told me that the theme would be farmhouse style, which I loved and was even the style of our new home to be built. I had another girlfriend who also offered, which was super sweet, and I jokingly allowed her to host one if I had a second. Micah was not impressed with the lack of response from his side of the family once the invite was sent on Facebook. He even sent a message on the family thread, and that was immediately dismissed, with his father bringing up Thanksgiving plans. I felt irritated as Micah's thunder was stolen from him. Baby showers don't come every year, and celebrating with his family was significant for him.

I finally told work about my pregnancy, and everyone was ecstatic! I was thinking about taking 6 months off starting January 1st, 2021. Hopefully, all would go as planned, and the baby wouldn't come too soon. One of my girlfriends reminded me she was three weeks early for both pregnancies! She predicted that since I am quite petite, I may be a bit early, too. Let's hope I finish my year without any interruptions.

The week of Labor Day, we booked a cabin for ourselves for a couple of nights and then another few nights with our friends. I noticed dirt and leaves on the floor when we arrived the first night. I was grossed out by looking at a completely unmade futon in the living room. The cleaning person didn't realize she had to come in that day. We were left to change our sheets and disinfect the cabin ourselves. We did end up receiving most of our money back. Micah didn't care about the fees totaling $150 that weren't refunded since we did stay for the two nights. We had a wonderful time with the Hood Canal in our front yard. We even gathered and shucked oysters for the first time and had a blast. We cooked it since I couldn't eat anything raw - they were the most delicious oysters I have ever had! Super fresh!

The next cabin we rented out was also on the canal just down the street. It was much larger and was right beside the state park. We observed a variety of wildlife during that stay - seals, elk, eagles, and even hummingbirds that flew to the windows to feast on the sugar water feeders (there was one that acted like such a jerk to the others and didn't want to share). When our friends arrived with their pups, it was a bit awkward because we weren't sure if we should wear masks inside so as not to give each other COVID, but we let go of the precautions and hoped for the best. Fear of contracting COVID was quite triggering, and we were all so bloody paranoid. It was as if we didn't know how to get back to normal, and when we tried, we felt like we were breaking the law. Apart from these initial dynamics, it was nice to be away from the city and have a change of pace from being locked up at home in isolation. However, the wildfires got out of hand all along the West Coast, and we had to lock ourselves up again due to the unhealthy air quality. If it wasn't airborne viruses, it was airborne particles. The year 2020 was not done with its wrath.

A couple of weeks after our cabin vacation, I was at week 23 and scheduled to do the fetal-echo ultrasound, which is a very detailed look at the heart. They look at every chamber, valve, artery, and all directions. Since I did IVF, the baby had a higher risk for heart defects. Thankfully, everything looked normal! This, again, was another one-hour appointment.

21. Twenty Four Weeks

At this point, I was cooking like an oven. I got all sweaty, even underneath my boobs, which I had never dealt with ever in my life. I felt hot and thirsty. My joints were sore due to water retention, and my heels ached when I walked. My sleep was interrupted in the middle of the night. It was uncomfy yet somewhat bearable. There were times of joy when the baby moved in my tummy, and Micah could also feel the movement. It was like the baby was playing with me as we would go back and forth, pushing on my tummy. Such endearing moments. Although, I wondered if he was just irritated being poked at.

We had our separate baby showers. The Cain family one was very nice at Luther Burbank Park on Mercer Island, near the water. Micah ordered banh mi and grabbed cupcakes and drinks. We tried to be as COVID-precautious as possible. The weekend after, I had my 2nd shower on my girlfriend's rooftop; it was the most magical event ever. It was way more than I could ever imagine, with lovely floral table decorations, a huge photo floral backdrop, swanky furniture, and all the divine details. I felt very supported and loved that afternoon. My girlfriend, T, knew how difficult my journey was. She wanted to go all out for me and she did. I am lucky to have her in my life, and she can empathize since she did IVF as well and had her own fertility journey. I also appreciated my other girlfriends who helped set up, cook, bring various supplies, and clean up. If I can be entirely honest, I had a couple of friends who did not quite understand how important this baby shower was to me. They just could not empathize with my fertility journey. Fortunately, and in general, my life is content. Thus, I can lend an ear, advise, and expend my energy and mental capacity on my girlfriends' life problems. I was hoping that because I usually ask for little, I could expect a bit more from my friends for my rare and special occasion. Of course, they love me, but where was the reciprocation in the friendship? I tried to be as understanding as possible, but then the other Gemini side of me was like, "WTF, lady? Didn't you realize that you should dress up for my baby shower when the invite explicitly said to dress up and be camera-ready? I mean, what part did you not understand?" One friend showed up in activewear and thought she had a great outfit. Smdh. Maybe the pandemic had a strange effect on some people, where social events weren't taken as seriously anymore, or they thought they could show up just the same for a non-virtual event because they worked in pajamas all day.

On the other hand, one other girlfriend dressed up like she was headed to the club. She looked hot, and I am so glad she dressed up, but it was a bit surprising. A couple of other gfs showed up late for who knows why, which put delays on setting up and organization; plus, there were a few other instances of odd behaviors, but I won't belabor this any longer.

We practiced proper COVID precautions for my shower, which was outdoors. All food was pre-packed in floral picnic bags, hand sanitizer was available, and there were no group activities where we would touch anything. We took some photos that may have seemed like we weren't being cautious, but my gfs wore their masks the entire time except for eating. They took their masks off for the pics just for that moment and tried not to breathe. These large group pics posted on social media caused misconceptions and family drama. My shower was the loveliest, and I was lucky I could even celebrate during this pandemic.

Sugar High

The Tuesday after my magical baby shower, I was scheduled for my blood glucose test, which was to decipher if I had gestational diabetes. The glucola drink I had to ingest had a very high sugar content. I was told the orange flavor was better than the fruit punch. At first, the drink wasn't bad tasting, but two-thirds of the way through, I felt a little gross and got a headache. I had to go to the lab for my blood test within an hour after finishing my concentrated sugar water. I wondered if this was as sweet as the hummingbird food I made.

I got a call for my results within a few days, and my glucose levels were at 197mg/dL. The normal range is 65-139mg/dL. Thus, I probably had gestational diabetes. The nurse suggested I do the 3-hour test, which required one to drink double the amount of glucola, and I was like,

"Excuse me?" I was not about to force feed myself and my baby more concentrated sugar water. So they said I could presume I had gestational diabetes and make appointments with the diabetes educator to control my blood sugar levels. So I opted for that. At my first appointment, the educator told me they shouldn't even have given me the option to take the second test because my levels were relatively high. I had already started testing my blood glucose levels, and it seemed okay, but what did I know? I was told that I most likely had some insulin resistance because of how my fasting levels looked, which were taken right after I woke up. I was still in denial about my gestational diabetes and thought, "Nah, I am fine." However, I was shown a figure showing how insulin resistance only increased as the pregnancy progressed, especially in the last few weeks. Some women have to go on meds a week before they deliver! I took this very seriously and adjusted my diet before this appointment. Exercise helped maintain healthy glucose levels, too.

Big Boobies and Babymoon Plans

For those deliberating on getting a boob job, get pregnant. Or, at least wait until after you breastfeed because you may be smaller than before, which was the circulating rumor. I was surprised to see that I went from a 34B to a 36C, and with milk, my boobs would be massive! I feel bad when I think about huge breasts, Dolly Parton comes to mind. I remember my mom would comment about her chest when she saw her on TV. She is obviously more than her figure and blonde hair. I was pretty impressed with her philanthropy work, especially in regards to COVID-19 vaccine research.

Speaking of COVID, Micah and I got antsy and booked another cabin trip for Thanksgiving weekend with his brother's family. I was curious about Hawaii and whether they would lift their 14-day quarantine when tourists arrived on the islands. Then on Oct.15th, all islands became open for vacationers with horrible cabin fever. If you took a COVID test 72 hours before your departure and were negative, you did not have to quarantine. I asked Micah if we should head to Kauai, and there was no hesitation. Being a scientist, I weighed the risks. Alaska Airlines mandated masks on the plane at all times except during eating/drinking, and that had to be "brief." All middle seats were blocked off for reservation to provide some "social distance". And, even though all tourists would have had a covid test within 72 hours, there was risk for

91

false negatives. Who knew if people were careful within that week as COVID took some time to showcase symptoms. Also, you could still spread it asymptomatically. The ventilation on the plane apparently was supreme, or at least I had to believe that. I was headed off of the mainland, which had thousands more cases than Kauai, which only had a few active cases. Thus, I was like YOLO. So we booked it for the end of October and would stay an entire week.

I still had my MVP Gold status with Alaska, and we got lucky to get upgraded to first class for free! I posted about this on FB, and the SIL who made the ridiculous comment about naming our son "Gosh" made another absurd comment. She asked if I had left Micah in coach. Firstly, I booked premium seats for both of us. Secondly, I wouldn't book with an airline that didn't upgrade my travel companion, either. Thirdly, if I had been the only one to get the complimentary upgrade, I was the one who actually earned it because I fly so much for work! I came back at her with a slightly snooty comment stating these facts with no further response on her end. Micah also commented that this was his first time in first class. I do feel she thinks the worst of me at times. Micah said his sister was not thinking in that manner, but he knows nothing about what actually goes on in the female brain and probably has not felt other micro-aggressions being a white male. Truly, his sisters don't know anything about me. They see what they see and paint their pictures. None have tried to get to know me, honestly. My respect and love for Micah is like none other. Plus, this sugar mama needs to take care of her sugar baby. Bahaaaaa! Believe it or not, he has become quite the princess, more snooty than me. My handsome, rugged ranger was not as rugged as he used to be, and it's all my fault!

Aloha

Planning for a COVID test within 72 hours of departure was stressful, especially if you tried to do the free or covered-by-insurance tests. Most testing sites were booked weeks in advance. Also, it wasn't just any COVID test; you had to schedule the specific ones listed on the Alaska Airlines COVID page. We did the rapid COVID test at Walgreens in Tacoma and received our results within an hour. It was so efficient. Luckily, we were both negative. We would have had to cancel the trip if we hadn't been negative. That would have been a mess to deal with. When we arrived at the airport, we were on the last flight of the day because of mechanical delays with other flights. Thus, the process was smooth and quick. The free first-class upgrade also ushered us to the front of the COVID check line.

The following day, we woke up to the most beautiful sunrise on the ocean, with palm trees swaying in the breeze. I booked a fabulous Airbnb, and the ocean front view never got tiresome. Kauai was abnormally hot and humid for early November, and we were on the third floor, so I was cooking like a mofo. There were fans but no air conditioner. I couldn't get cooler during the day or at night before bed. Essentially, I was stripped down to my underwear on the bed while using a damp face cloth to continuously wipe my arms and legs while the fan was aimed straight at me. I felt like an overheated beached whale. Luckily, it was the only price I had to pay to be in paradise. What was more important was staying COVID-free.

The fresh tropical fruit, real vitamin D, and warm ocean waters blessed our babymoon. Of course, my darling IG husband got straight to work and snapped a bunch of baby bump photos on the beaches of Kauai.

Obsessed

I was fascinated with the baby's movements because they had become much more substantial. I watched my tummy and poked back when I felt a poke. He sometimes curled up on one side of my ribs, which was uncomfortable. His motions could be quite powerful, almost as if he wanted to escape my tummy already. I watched a video indicating that at 32 weeks, the baby was about 4 pounds and close to 17 inches long; thus, they wanted to stretch out since they were so confined. This made total sense because he would sit his rump to one side and make my tummy look all misshapen. It was humorous at times when I felt like he was taking his elbow or hand and smearing it along the wall of my stomach. Micah was also mesmerized and shocked when he felt this with his hand.

My gestational diabetes seemed to be under control, and when I felt a little icky from insulin resistance, I used our stairs to do some exercise, and this helped bring down my glucose levels. Just recently, I did not feel as hungry as I had expected at this time, and it was nice not to have to feel like I had to eat immediately at every moment. Every bit of pregnancy was utterly exhausting.

I began my nesting activities for the baby's arrival. I cleaned out three drawers to make room for baby clothes and supplies. We debated getting a changing table with drawers but had no space. Our friends said we shouldn't limit ourselves to just one room to change the baby. Thus, we opted for a changing pad for downstairs, and we used our bed upstairs with a waterproof quilted liner and toted around our felt diaper caddy. Convenience and free space took precedence.

<u>Vlogs Published</u>

I released my fertility vlogs to the public on YouTube. I began recording right before I started my IVF cycle to document and share my journey. The responses from other mothers undergoing IVF were touching. Most of these moms had to go through multiple rounds of IVF before having a successful pregnancy. Complications such as endometritis (inflammation of the inner lining of the uterus), inadequate progesterone hormone levels, and multiple egg retrievals were mentioned. Just thinking about what these women went through was draining. Imagine the stress and anxiety they had to carry with them while trying to remain positive and hopeful all the while. It was pretty remarkable, all of it.

Reproduction and fertility are often not spoken of outwardly or publicly. Some people are uncomfortable sharing because they think it is private and may be embarrassed about their experiences trying to conceive. Through my vlogs, I hoped to open up those closed channels so that women could speak about their journeys in order to have an open dialogue. Most women go through it alone and don't have to. I feel much support is needed, especially for those who have miscarried. Many times, women blame themselves, feel guilty, and ashamed. This needs to change, and we need more education and information from all parties involved, including from society.

Lena Dunham (loved Girls btw) had an article published in the December 2020 issue of Harper's Magazine titled "False Labor." I read a few opinion pieces on how betrayed and insulted some felt about the snide/sarcastic comments Lena made regarding certain fertility support groups. (Check out IVF Warrior on Instagram. They even have an Etsy.)

After I read the piece, I didn't see a villain but a hurt girl who had her childhood dreams crushed because of her reproductive biology. Sure, she spoke about how disgusted she was with white, privileged women who made up the majority of these support groups while ironically being a white, privileged woman herself for those who may not be familiar with her. (I do commend her on using her platform though for this.) She eloquently raged about her frustrations with the world and ranted that life was completely unfair. Following that piece, there were more articles published about how traumatic her reproductive journey was and how IVF destroyed her body, which resulted in one functioning ovary left with the hope of harvesting viable eggs. This resulted in more crushing news that her eggs were not adequate. Adoption would be her only option.

First thing this morning, I received a message from an acquaintance congratulating me and then mentioning that her gf had two failed IVF cycles. I truly felt for this woman and all women who were struggling with their reproduction. Most feel helpless and disappointed that the organs they were born with were not operating correctly, no matter how hard they try. I gave some tips and the link to my vlog if her gf was interested. I hoped my vlogs resonated with those on their fertility journey and provided helpful tips and advice.

I knew two women who planned to do egg retrievals in the winter who were both in their mid thirties. Friend #1 was devastated when she learned of her AMH levels, which were very low (~0.2). Friend #2 told me her results, which were quite exceptional (3.89). I hoped both would have successful egg retrievals, but I worried about #1. She became pregnant before, but unfortunately, that ended in miscarriage right after the first trimester. I was sure all the stress from her divorce, the pandemic, career, and life took a toll on her graceful body. I told her she should rest and do acupuncture to get her body ready, but I don't think she listened. I advised her to gain some weight and modify her diet. She has a new partner now and is thinking of fertilizing the embryos and transferring them immediately, which I thought was wise given her situation. #2 gained some weight during the last half year, which I thought was positive for her retrieval. She felt sad because she was doing this without a partner. Life doesn't always happen the exact way we want it. Thus, we must forge our paths and take control of our destinies.

There is nothing more powerful than your autonomy and taking action to build the life you want to live.

22. Happy COVID Christmas

Week 36 came so quickly. I tried to relax as much as possible (basically Netflix binging), eat well, exercise on my stairs, complete my work tasks (because of preggy brain, I found myself being relatively slow), educate myself on everything and anything baby-related, do nesting activities, and finish my magazine project Vietology... we are on Facebook and Instagram (@viet.ology).

We celebrated our COVID Christmas in isolation with our pups and steamed some live Dungeness crab. America was #1 for COVID cases and deaths for the entire world. The surges continued, and hospitals were at capacity in some states. Millions of Americans traveled out of state for Thanksgiving and Christmas, even with warnings about the dangers of intermixing households. But your freedom and liberties are more important than keeping a pandemic at bay, right? Families shouldn't have celebrated together unless all members isolated themselves for at least 7-10 days. I couldn't trust my in-laws because they assembled with their Mormon church where most, if not all, did not believe in social distancing. What was remarkable was that my father-in-law (FIL), who is a Republican and had stage IV lung cancer, could die if he got COVID and became severely ill. A SIL asked me if I would allow Micah's father and stepmother to see the baby, and I replied that no one would see the baby during this pandemic. I was not risking my baby's health, period. One of my other SILs (I have five) asked if anyone would be willing to quarantine themselves and help us once the baby was here; the answer was an absolute no. I mean, who had the luxury of helping us at that moment? I suppose I could have hired a doula, but I would have to trust that this person was COVID-free and would remain that way for her time with us. Honestly, I never had anyone in mind to help us at all, only our mothers if they were still alive. This baby was our responsibility, and we must work together as a family. I don't know how single mothers do it; I am sure they always hear that. They are my heroes.

I had my 36-week ultrasound, and it was great to see the baby, although because his head was so low in my cervix, we couldn't get a sweet profile shot. Instead, I got a gorgeous clear shot of his spine. He was a healthy 6 lb 7oz baby in the 57th percentile, with a strong heartbeat, and was positioned correctly for birth. That was all that mattered. This was also the first week for the non-stress test (NST) for the baby, where I was hooked up to an ultrasound that would capture the baby's movements and heartbeat. The only images produced were waves and peaks, akin to a lie detector test. Every time I felt the baby move, I pressed the button to indicate movement and watched the machine create a peak, which recorded my baby's increased heart rate. The NST lasted twenty minutes and was designed to ensure the baby was doing well and getting enough oxygen. My OBGYN prescribed it for me because of my advanced maternal age and gestational diabetes. What was interesting about my gestational diabetes was that I thought it would get worse as I went further into my pregnancy. Since it has been totally under control, I become less affected by insulin intolerance. My fasting levels were under 95mg/dL each morning, and after I ate, my glucose levels were stable, unlike before when I would have pretty dramatic drops or increases.

This week, I also finished the last blood testing card for the ASPIRE study, which followed women through their pandemic pregnancy. I look forward to the results. Also, I recently joined their private FB group and found two other women with the same due date as me, which was incredible!

My tummy felt so huge by now, and the baby liked to stick his butt out so far that it deformed my belly, making me uncomfortable. The baby was plumping up and taking more space than I could give. I felt better as the week progressed, and my skin stretched out more. Sleeping was somewhat uncomfortable as my left hip was sore, and the baby liked to push on my bladder really well in the middle of the night. He even shifted over to the left side for some reason, and my left ribs were probably slightly bruised. Baby's hiccups were quite strong now, too, because he was so big.

I began a few new routines at 36 weeks: drinking raspberry leaf tea (to help with uterine health and cervical effacement), eating three organic Medjool dates a day (apparently, this helps with certain hormone levels), taking two primrose capsules orally and inserting one vaginally in the evening (helps with softening of the cervix), and perineum stretching. This was Micah's duty every evening for 10 minutes. He'd stretch my vagina so that I could have a gaping hole and not tear. The perineum stretching was interesting. I'd sit back on the couch spread eagle and watch TV while Micah lubed his fingers to stretch the muscle. At first, I had to breathe and relax to release that tension. The first time we did this exercise, it hurt a lot when Micah took his fingers out. It felt like he was pulling the tissues of my vagina wall off. Thus, I highly recommend lubricant. We also added some vitamin E oil. If I ended up having a C-section, this was all in vain, but at least I was prepared!

For Christmas, the most important gift I received was Micah's genetic testing to reveal his ethnicity breakdown. The results from CRI Genetics showcased that he is 33% German, 24% Italian, 13% British, 11% Southern, Central Slavic, 9% French, and 8% Scandinavian. We were pretty surprised by the Italian portion and had no clue. I was super glad he did it! I did 23andMe and Ancestry DNA last Christmas, and I am mainly Vietnamese and some Chinese.

38 Weeks

So, any day now. Micah gave me "permission" to have my baby today at 38 weeks old because our close friends were returning from the cabin and could take care of our crazy shiba puppy, Tomtom, a black & tan foofer. Our neighbors would take Yuki, our older orange shiba, who is a breeze. I wanted my baby to stay inside for another week for more development and growth. At my last appointment, I was given a one-pager on induction, which sounded horrid. I hoped that my pregnancy would not result in any of the methods listed, which sounded risky, uncomfortable, and unnatural. Here are some of the methods (mayoclinic.org):

Ripening of the cervix using synthetic prostaglandins placed inside the vagina. They may want to stick an inflatable balloon into your cervix and fill it with saline to help ripen the cervix.

Rupturing of the amniotic sac with a plastic hook.

Use of intravenous medication with oxytocin (Pitocin), which causes the uterus to contract

All of these procedures came with risks, such as failed induction, low heart rate, infection, uterine rupture, and increased risk of severe bleeding after delivery. Sounds wonderful, ya? Micah reminded me of some pressure points he could press on when the time came. Apparently, some pre-natal massages can also jump-start birth.

I was getting up in the middle of the night and usually a bit hungry, so I'd have a snack and, in my boredom, post things on social media at 4 am, which people may have found odd if they noticed the time stamp. I mean, my network needed to know the connection between vitamin D deficiency and the risk of COVID infection, right? And, that I would prefer bitcoin as a push present rather than designer bags and diamond rings. Some women didn't know what a push present was, which surprised me. Essentially, it's a lavish gift for the mother-to-be because she had a foreign body within her own body for approximately 10 whole months, had to push a baby out of her vagina (or have a C-section), and deserves the bloody world for it. I think this is something rich people thought of because I became aware of this practice when I was with my ex, whose sister received luxurious gifts after pushing out a few daughters. I was all for this type of showcase of gratification. Truly, the gifts were the least you could do for a mummy who sacrificed her own well-being for her offspring.

Snip Snip?

So I asked my gfs who had boys whether they had their sons circumcised or not. The majority did. I had a couple gfs say they wouldn't do it again, and another gf said she regretted not having it done. While these days, circumcision is more of an aesthetic choice, I do think that it seems more hygienic in general. I mean, boys are dirty, and gross gunk can get stuck in the folds of the skin. Micah recently watched a YT video on an adult male who had to get circumcised in his 20s because of current fungal infections. This man mentioned that sex was more pleasurable with the foreskin, but eventually, he got used to it. If a baby was circumcised from the start, he wouldn't know any better.

Micah was unsure if he wanted to take that away from his son. On the other hand, not having foreskin apparently makes you last longer in bed. It really was a toss up and at first we thought we would have our boy circumcised.

23. Did It Happen Yet?

So it seemed that baby Dang-Cain wanted to cook in mummy's tummy longer. I was going to be 40 weeks in two days. I had an appointment the day before with my OBGYN. After checking the amniotic fluid via ultrasound and sticking her fingers up my vagina to get a good feel of my cervix, we decided to schedule an induction for the evening of next Tuesday for next-day delivery. They wanted to prepare and "ripen" my cervix by thinning it out, and then, if no contractions occurred, they'd give me oxytocin to jump-start uterine contractions. My doctor sensed that I was a bit hesitant about the induction, but I truly wanted what was best for my baby. The amniotic fluid was low-normal, and at first, she was concerned about my baby.

When I asked if I should have an induction earlier, she said no. So that wasn't very clear. I mean, were you concerned or not concerned? I also have to add that I had my shoes on while lying on the table, and when she switched from the ultrasound to check my cervix, she grabbed my foot to place on the stirrups and continued to lube up and stick that same gloved hand up my cervix. It all occurred so quickly, and I was shocked that she thought it was hygienic enough to touch my shoe and then stick her hand up my vagina. The funny thing was that I felt I should have slipped my shoes off, which I usually did, but I kept them on that day for some reason. Maybe it was because I wasn't wearing any socks. Micah was astonished that I didn't say anything, and I was like, if she were about to deliver my baby, I would prefer not to make it even more awkward between us. I prayed I wouldn't get some gross infection, which was highly unlikely as the vagina can keep itself clean reasonably well.

The non-stress tests came out fine, which was reassuring. The baby seemed to be acting normal. I did have moments where, if I hadn't felt him for a little bit, I feared the worst. He was a fairly active baby, so it freaked me out when he went to sleep and rested. I assumed he had become much plumper because my tummy itched, and I was getting some stretch marks around my belly button. I was so lucky up until now with my skin. I worked hard to moisturize it and noticed some petechiae, little red dots under the skin that look like tiny speckles of internal bleeding. I leveled up, grabbed the vitamin E in my cupboard, and began massaging that on my tummy. Hopefully, that would alleviate some stretching, although I will probably have some marks for life. Women have to suffer for their babies quite a bit, physically and mentally. And, speaking of suffering, my lower back ached from all the front belly weight. Sitting and sleeping became uncomfortable, bowel movements were difficult, and I waddled and walked quite slowly. Ah, pregnancy was such a beautiful thing. I used an exercise ball to sit on and did figure 8's, one technique for naturally inducing if the baby was in the correct position. I found it alleviated some back pelvic discomfort, too. Micah began to press on specific pressure points that may also help induce them. I scheduled a massage and an acupuncture appointment, thinking that would do the trick. Micah even had a sex session scheduled. I wondered how that would turn out at 10 months pregnant.

I Think Something Is Happening

I made it up to my last day of work before maternity leave. My co-workers were impressed that the baby didn't want to come out of his comfy little nest and joked about how it got the memo about the pandemic and other civil unrest in America. I had my massage midday, and the therapist, a brand new graduate, researched pressure points before working on me. After my session, I was skeptical of this newbie but was impressed by her technique. She wished me luck and hoped my water would break soon. Later that afternoon, around 5 pm, I took a nap. I roused at about 6 pm and felt a pop in my vaginal area and then noticed some fluid gushing out. I checked my underwear and saw some pinkish/red discharge and decided it was my mucous plug ejecting itself. Then, the contractions came, and I began timing/recording them. Each became more painful within the hour, and I knew Micah should get ready to leave. He called the OBGYN office, and they told me to come in as my contractions seemed to be occurring every 5-6 minutes or so quite regularly. Before we got to the hospital, we had to drop our two dogs off at their aunt and uncle's, which was only a few minutes away from the hospital. I could barely say bye to the dogs as the contractions became less bearable as time passed. Micah reminded me to breathe deeply, and that helped.

Once we arrived at the hospital, I was offered a wheelchair and gladly took it. Labor and delivery was on the 5th floor, and after check-in, we were guided to an examination room, where we waited for the nurse. I heard a woman moaning in pain down the hall. Micah hoped I wouldn't notice, but you had to be deaf not to notice it. A friendly nurse finally arrived and wanted to check out my cervix.

"You're about five centimeters dilated already. We will get you into a delivery room soon. Do you want an epidural? If so, this would be the right time."

"Yes, please!"

Micah and I were both astonished at how quickly everything was moving. My contractions continued to become more intense. Micah coached me through them with deep breathing. Within 10 minutes of seeing the first nurse, a second nurse escorted me to the delivery room. His name was Timothy, and he would be assisting with the labor and delivery. I was not used to male health professionals seeing my private parts, but thankfully, I got over it quickly as the ones I encountered were very professional. Plus, I had no say in the matter as a baby was about to be ejected from my body soon. It was possible that Timothy was not heterosexual, which made me more comfortable with him because there would be no creep factor. He also had a very tender and caring bedside manner, which I greatly appreciated.

I was rolled into the delivery room and couldn't wait for the bloody epidural. Timothy had to get an IV into my veins and couldn't seem to get a proper poke on the first, second, and third try. He even had to get a vein finder using some red laser light thingy. Finally, they gave up on my forearm and just used the presentable vein in the crook of my elbow, which was more irritating for the patient. Micah was a bit flabbergasted at all the pokes to my poor arm, but I had barely noticed since my contracting uterus was sending vibrations of sheer pain throughout my body. The anesthesiologist finally arrived and explained what he would be doing while placing my epidural. He was such a master I didn't feel anything and even had a button I could press to add more drugs to my spine if needed. It was so nice to feel less pain with my contractions. Timothy was quite impressed at my ability to tolerate the pain. I do believe my threshold is quite high.

A petite woman came in and introduced herself as my delivery doc. Most women assume their OBGYN will deliver their baby, but I don't think that is usually the case, especially for midnight deliveries. Dr. T reminded me of the actress Leslie Mann. We discussed if I had a birthing plan, and I said whatever it took to get the baby out in the most efficient and safest ways. She even allowed me to rest for a few hours before delivery. I never thought I would be able to take a nap before I pushed my baby out. What a luxury! Epidurals are the best, and I highly recommend them if you are on the fence. I actually cannot believe I thought I should ever go without one to be honest.

The delivery room was spacious and quite lovely to be in. The ambiance was serene with the dimmed lights, and most of the time, it was just Timothy, Micah, and me. It was 11:45 pm, and Dr. T came by to tell me to start pushing. She left and would be back later to check on the progress. My contractions were being monitored, but I could tell when they would be coming on before the machine recorded the peak. Timothy coached me the whole way through, and I was instructed to push like I was pooping for two rounds of counts to ten. It wasn't easy to push for ten counts because I would lose my breath and stamina. After each round of pushing, I became so ill I ralphed in the green plastic bag given to me. The retching was so intense in my stomach, as if I had a terrible case of food poisoning. I thought it may have been side effects of the epidural, but it was probably just the act of giving birth itself. Timothy continued to provide me with cold, damp face cloths to wipe my mouth and place on my hot head. Initially, my feet were placed on a bar, and I was to grab behind my knees, pull myself up as if doing crunches, and push simultaneously. At one point, my leg fell off the bar that my foot was placed on, and Micah and the nurse looked in horror at my dangling leg. The amount of work delivery requires is ridiculously strenuous. Pregnant people are effin' warriors.

After a couple of hours of pushing, Dr. T came to check on me and told me to push down and up or to at least visualize this motion since the birth canal wasn't a straight shot out, so it was kind of like the bottom part of the letter C. My legs were placed in large plastic stirrups, and they put a bar in front of me with a sheet to use as a pull. I was doing half-body pull-ups with each contraction. Timothy continued to monitor the baby's heartbeat. They could see his head, but delivery was taking a while. Dr. T said if the baby's heartbeat slowed at all, we would have to do a C-section. I definitely would rather have a vaginal birth, but I would do whatever it took to have a safe delivery.

Also, I did not want to end up like other mums I knew who refused a C-section and put themselves in unnecessary lengthy delivery (like 24-30 hours) and then ended up doing a C-section anyway. We kept on. Every 8-10 minutes, I felt the contractions coming, would push for two counts of ten, ralph, and then was knocked out until the next contraction. Dr. T even added petocin to my IV to have the contractions come more regularly, but that didn't help so much. It was almost 4 am, and the baby was finally coming out of my vagina at a quicker pace. Micah got my phone ready to record. He continued to give me words of affirmation, which helped quite a bit since I had no idea how I was doing. I needed all the encouragement I could get. Dr. T was with us for the last hour or so as she probably had no other deliveries to tend to. She was spreading my labia to make room for the baby's head that had been crowning. Micah said the baby's head would push out more each time but then retract. I made a huge push, and I heard Dr. T exclaim that the baby was coming out with the next one. I gave it my all on the next contraction and out popped little Tobin at 4:01 am. Timothy immediately placed him on my chest and wiped him down. Completely exhausted, I praised my baby like he was a little puppy. His eyes were wide open straight out of the birth canal. It was an incredible sight.

We spent a few more hours in the delivery room while I recovered. Timothy's shift was over, and he almost didn't want to leave us. I think he wanted to be friends with us. It was sweet. Another nurse came in to empty my bladder with a catheter and noted that my vagina was highly inflamed, so she got an ice pack. I had to get a catheter placed up my urethra twice to drain my bladder. The second time, the epidural was wearing off, so I felt a little bit of pain. My bladder needed to be drained immediately, according to the nurse. When it was time to relocate to the recovery room, I could not get up at all, so they wheeled me down to the floor below in a bed. The new room was much smaller and older looking. They probably didn't want patients to stay long, so they gave you a room you would rather not be in. It was such a pity compared to the lovely delivery room. We had nurses check on us every few hours, and I had to manually stimulate for colostrum to come out of my boobs, which was difficult since I had no idea what I was doing. The nurses helped a lot and did a better job of hand expressing.

Colostrum is a sticky liquid that is greenish brown at first. I tried to get Tobin to latch on, but that was something to be learned as the days went by. On the first attempt, he damaged my right nipple, and some tissue broke out from my skin. It was somewhat disturbing. I was given lanolin and hydrogel nipple covers to aid in healing. I was also taught how to use a nipple shield while feeding since my nipples were a bit short, and for the baby to latch correctly, he needed to be stimulated by the soft palate. Other mums had shared how breastfeeding was challenging, but I never knew how much work it would entail.

When we left the hospital after being there for less than 48 hours, it felt like we were in another dimension or abducted by aliens. The world outside felt like it had paused while we were gone. We were probably delirious. Bringing home this newborn baby was surreal.

24. New Parent Life

The COVID-19 vaccine became available for the general public in January of 2021, only if there was a vaccine surplus since they didn't want any to go to waste. Once the vaccine thawed, it had to be used within a certain number of hours. We received a text from my pharmacist girlfriend in the middle of the night asking us to head to Seattle Central College if we wanted our first shot. So we grabbed our sleeping two-week-old and were on our way. It felt as if we were privy to some magical antidote since the vaccines were only available for frontline healthcare workers, seniors, and high-risk individuals. The Moderna mRNA produced copies of spike protein in our system, and the side effects impeded our new parent duties even more. It was worth it, though, because I would be transferring protective COVID-19 antibodies to my baby via breast milk, which would be the first steps in building up his immune system.

The first few months were rough. I was a slave to my baby and the breast pump. I signed up for a lactation consultation two weeks after I delivered, which was helpful. As Tobin's head grew, he became more efficient at latching on properly, and my nipples became accustomed to breastfeeding. I no longer needed to use the nipple shield after a month, and I still applied the lanolin or nipple butter after each feeding to protect my skin. Pumping was so much work, which I did after every feeding to stimulate more milk production, and I detested it so much. It felt like an awful chore I had to do numerous times daily. It didn't hurt; it was just irritating that I had to do another activity with my boobs after already breastfeeding my baby when all I wanted to do was just rest. My pelvic floor took at least 6 weeks to recover as it was very delicate the first 2 weeks and felt like it was going to fall out of my body. The nurse gave me a velcro belly band, adding more abdominal support and allowing me to walk around more easily. I began getting massages again as I developed some back and hip soreness. It had been 2.5 months, and time went by quickly due to the repetition of routines and constant care. I was a robot trying to keep this tiny human alive. The most important activity, besides getting a few winks of sleep in, was getting fed properly. We were so grateful for our friends and family who dropped food off for us. I was told to sleep while the baby slept, but that was tough because I had chores that needed to be done. Luckily, our baby enjoyed sleeping, and by about a month, he had slept through the night for about 6-8 hours.

Don't Breathe On or Come Near My Baby!

Navigating this pandemic was a struggle, especially with Micah's family. Most people do not understand proper disinfection and how to prevent transmission of viruses to other people. No matter how I said it or spelled it out, it was difficult for people to comprehend that I didn't want them near my baby during the pandemic. Family members especially thought they had certain access and privileges because they were family. Even if I told them not to kiss the baby, they still did because their baby fever so blinded them. To give a non-pandemic example, I was telling my SIL to stop rocking the baby so vigorously, and even though she heard this, she continued, and the baby barfed just like I said he would. I had to tell both my SILs to stop rocking the baby so much after eating, and it was as if I was speaking a foreign language. The aggravation, my god.

I may have forgotten to mention that the summer I was pregnant, Micah and I decided to put a deposit down on a new development just east of Seattle. So what that meant was we needed to sell our townhouse, which was in the Columbia City area. The housing market was on fire for sellers. Supply was low and demand was high - bidding wars were becoming insane. Thus, while caring for a newborn, we decided to get rid of all our furniture, pack everything we didn't need in storage, and live like nomads with our two Shiba Inus. I was so exhausted that I almost couldn't bring myself to pack up all of my art, which consisted of 5x4 ft pieces. I was almost in tears because I could not get up off the floor. We had no couch because we had sold it. Never had I ever felt this type of weariness. I was depleted physically and mentally. My hormones were off the charts, I was still recovering from delivery, and all of my energy was going towards producing breast milk. What would have normally taken two grown adults sans baby to do in a week took us two. But we cleared it out, and our realtor took care of the rest.

It was the end of March 2021, and since we were homeless, Micah and I decided to move in with his father and his wife for a month to spend time with him as he had stage 4 lung cancer. He was a non-smoker, by the way. We were under the suspicion that his cancer was the cause of the J&J talcum powder that contained asbestos he had used religiously for years.

Our polite requests were pretty simple: to not have people come into the house and for them to try not to meet with their friends indoors. Both rules were broken. Because my FIL and his wife are Mormon, there are plenty of occasions to meet and greet. Weekly dinner gatherings began outside but ended up inside because of high winds, blessings before surgery, and Easter, to name a few. We had our rules thrown back in our faces because we ate out at restaurants that would follow COVID procedures and were in actual controlled environments. We were told that we were being hypocritical. While it was possible that airborne virus exposure could occur within a restaurant even while being socially distant at 25% capacity, and if air circulation was poor, at least no one was trying to be in our baby's bubble. My in-laws would attend gatherings in someone's house with around 15 people wearing no masks.

Folks also did not understand or forgot that babies must build their immune systems up, which takes time. Yes, there may be some antibodies that are passed in utero and even via breastfeeding, but we didn't know to what extent our baby was protected. And, even if he was fully protected, why would we want to risk exposure by not being vaccinated? My FIL apparently could not get a COVID-19 vaccine due to his cancer treatments, but as for his wife, she had no excuse. They are Mormon AND Republican. Tucker Carlson was the true expert and only stated facts. Speaking of my step-MIL, on day two of being in their household, I already felt unwelcomed. I placed my suitcase in her barely used arts & crafts room, and when we came home from dinner, I found a note on the door to take my stuff out because this was her room. The note also indicated that we should not put food or water on the broken ping-pong table, the same table that was going to be tossed when they decided to sell the house. We only had the luxury of having the tiniest counter space to put our food-related items in their expansive kitchen. It

110

was also really fun to go to the garage and access the fridge where we had to store our food so it could be separated from theirs within the kitchen. This was family. I was already hormonal and exhausted, and having to deal with these rules and restrictions drove me even more mad. This seemed like the worst idea in the world, but I had to grin and bear it because Micah's father's life expectancy was unpredictable.

Micah and I argued about the whole charade because I posted it on social media. His siblings saw it and were appalled at my display of the family dynamics. I had many validating comments from my network, which was gratifying. It wasn't like I had an actual bond with my step-MIL who wanted to be called grandma yet treated immediate family like third-class citizens. There was no actual relationship to maintain, and there were just way too many rules coming in as "family." Going back to me and Micah, he was distraught and nervous his father would get wind of this post, making him sick to his stomach. He thought his father would find it ungrateful and kick us out. I was willing to take those chances because the whole thing was ludicrous, and my FIL should realize a few things before he passes. Yet, I was in no mood to sit down and talk about it because I didn't expect them to change, and they won't ever change. Thus, it was moot even to bring it up unless they found out. This was the first time I feared that Micah would see me in a different light or love me less. He thought I was reckless and could not understand my need to post it on FB. He kept saying, "I would never do that," and I replied, "Yes, and I am not you." I was being silenced if I couldn't express my grievances in my manner. I don't do well with censorship. It took about a week or so for Micah to let this go, and he felt better after I blocked his family from this one post.

This was probably the sixth biggest fight we ever had. Out of the ten years we had been together, I could count the hugest fights that have occurred on one hand. These dynamics differed from those in my previous relationships, where a big blowout fight was more common. It all came down to maturity and communication. Both of them were at the young adulthood stage, along with my exes. Thus, there was so much growth and development to be had. Things were fine for a few weeks after that debacle, and we decided to stay one more week after his father's lung procedure.

We're Leaving. Now.

The evening before my FIL had his surgery, two Mormons with no masks came into the house to do a blessing. I was upstairs but glanced down below and noticed this atrocity. Micah verified this when he went down with the baby to say hi. I was livid that my FIL would break his promise of having people over, and if he wanted them to come, we could have left the house, but we didn't know they wouldn't be wearing masks. The following morning, I told Micah that we were leaving. His father had already gone to the hospital for his surgery, so there was no awkward confrontation. He told his stepmom some lie about work for the early departure. It was probably for the best that he didn't tell the truth, but it boggled my mind how some people found it challenging to be honest. Perhaps for the sake of being less awkward, I suppose. So many family dramas occur because people aren't being forthright. Either way, it didn't matter, I guess, because we were leaving. It took half a day for us to get adequately packed up with the baby and two dogs. We had to drive separately since we had both cars with us. Fortunately and miraculously, baby Tobin slept for the whole 3.5-hour drive back. Maybe there was comfort in being sandwiched between the dogs. If I had to stay out in eastern Washington another week, I would have completely lost it. There were so many emotions swirling in my head. I was out of my element, had no actual home where I could just be comfortable, was on COVID high-alert mode for my baby, and my hormones were wack. It was a circus.

Dumping Milk at D-land

One of my girlfriends and I have the same birthday. We girls went to Disneyland to celebrate and had a blast. I never thought I would enjoy myself at D-land, but I did. It was the first time I would be away from my baby! The plan was to stay for three nights. Micah had his sister to help out if needed since she lived upstairs. We rented out her basement Airbnb for the next three months while we waited for our house to be built.

I brought a Haakaa manual breast pump with me, which I hadn't ever used before. It sucked (no pun intended) and was not efficient like my Spectra pump at home. This product was better for those mums with breast milk that gushed out non-stop. It wasn't doing the job, and my boobs were swollen with milk. While at D-land, I went into a washroom with a paper cup to try to hand-squeeze milk out. My boobs were weighing me down, literally, and I couldn't fully enjoy my time at the happiest place on earth. Hand expressing was not working; I probably only got a few squirts. I feared that my ducts would become blocked. I couldn't stand it anymore and was missing my baby, so I found an earlier flight out the day before I was supposed to leave. Somehow, this flight was cheaper, and I got some money back for switching. My gf was a bit disappointed, but eight other girls were there to continue the birthday weekend celebrations. Micah was surprised I came home early. I couldn't wait to breastfeed! My boobs were about to explode.

25. Turning 40 in the Era of COVID

I didn't think I would do anything for my 40th since we were still in the pandemic, and most restaurants weren't doing large parties. I saw an IG post from a friend who had a loft space at Melrose Market in Capitol Hill, and she was allowing gatherings. So, a few weeks before my birthday, I decided to have a party. Only three people were not vaccinated at my party, and I didn't know they weren't vaccinated before they arrived. They didn't bother wearing their masks. I should have insisted they wear them, but I was trying to have a good time with my friends, and I didn't want to be that person, even though I should have been that person. I mean, my party, my rules, plus my baby was present. At this moment during the pandemic, cases were dramatically low, and the majority of Washingtonians had at least one shot. Delta was still the variant circulating, but things seemed to be getting better during the summer of 2021. This was our first big celebration in over a year with all our friends. No one got COVID at my party, thank goodness. I had a wonderful time. Micah even got me a beautiful cake in the shape of a baby grand because that was exactly what he got me in real life for our new dream house. I was a happy birthday girl and very grateful for my life.

Please Don't Breathe on My Baby. Part II.

One of my friends invited me to her swanky rooftop for an intimate birthday pre-game party. She told me there would be food and drinks, and it would be grand. The caveat was that it was being held for this social butterfly in Seattle, who loved to be the center of attention and thought he should be invited to every party. This same dude cried to my girlfriend about not being invited to my intimate 40th birthday. This person didn't think I liked him, but I couldn't give a fuh. I had my own life and close friends to worry about. Why would I care about acquaintances I found not genuine and quite tactical in their social maneuvers? Oh, I forgot to add that he had been in love with one of my best friends since day one, and she friend-zoned him so hard that he was too scared to confess his love. It was pretty comical, and I felt terrible for the guy. So, after much PR talk and buttering, I agree to attend this intimate, classy soiree.

Per the invite request, Micah, myself, and Tobin arrived looking super sweet in mainly white. I saw several folks, but my girlfriend was nowhere in sight. She was still working because when you work for Amazon, you never stop working. Ever. I was annoyed and unsurprised. I then had to chat it up with the birthday boy and his crew, which was fine. What wasn't fine was that this intimate, classy soiree was casual, and we were eating stale Vietnamese food. Essentially, my gf, who was supposed to be the host, was nowhere in sight; it was a complete waste of my time.

I was bamboozled and will never attend any event related to this birthday boy who even dared to say he "missed" my birthday party. WTF? You weren't invited, bruh! And get this—My other gf (the one who friend-zoned the birthday boy) told me the day after the event that no one in that group was vaccinated. I was mortified and yelled at the "host" (my gf) via text. Thank goodness I didn't let anyone hold my baby. I had walked into a room full of anti-vaxxers and had no clue. I should have begun all my conversations by asking, "What are your feelings on COVID shots?" I was upset at myself for not being more careful and should not have agreed to come to appease my gf, who was overly concerned about PR and networking.

Killing It

I was excited to get back to work. I needed something else to do besides take care of my baby. Feeling productive in my career is essential to my well-being, I've come to realize. I received messages from colleagues who said they missed me, and it felt good to be valued. During my leave, one of my colleagues, who I referred to the company, became my manager. My previous manager received a promotion. At first, there was annoying micromanagement, but as the months went on and the trust grew, I quickly became the team's star. My new manager praised me to the higher-ups and even got me another raise. Going on maternity leave was the best thing that ever happened to me because I came back blazing! My colleagues had much heavy lifting to do because the team was slim. They were probably burnt out and happy I was back. I was coming up on my fifth year with the company, and my director was working on promoting me to a higher level. That fiscal year was one of my most productive, and I had various development opportunities.

Oh, I forgot to mention that I sold two of my original 4ft x 4ft paintings in April of 2022. People still loved my art! Yay! The person who purchased the pieces had my card from a while back and found it. He had seen my art in a café previously and didn't even need to look at the paintings in person to solidify the deal, which was pretty incredible. Most folks want to see it up close and inspect it. He just trusted his gut, I guess. My gf joined me when I dropped them off at his place for safety reasons. His wife was also there, which was reassuring, but who knows these days. People can be crazy. It was rewarding to speak to customers during the transaction; they were mesmerized when they saw the pieces IRL (in real life). I sold these two paintings, and I still miss them. When my paintings leave my ownership, a wisp of my spirit accompanies it.

Superspreader Party

Taking a COVID test is just like taking a pregnancy test (different sampling method, of course - one is pee on a stick, the other snot swab), except you don't want it to be positive!! And, when you see that second purple line, it's like, eff my life!

So, I finally got COVID in May of 2022. Barely anyone wore a mask, and it was a free-for-all. The ridiculous part was that I got it at an event I was hosting! I got it there or right before it; there was no way of knowing. We probably all should have taken a test the morning of, which, might I add, was Friday the 13th. I consider that a lucky day because I loathe and face superstitions head-on. So I had a magazine launch party for Vietology, my published baby. I probably forgot to mention that while caring for my newborn, I also continued to have bi-weekly meetings with my team to produce a final product for our first issue, which was on Women & the Arts. Our primary mission was to highlight inspirational Vietnamese individuals. At max, there were probably close to 30-40 folks at peak time. It was indoors, and only one attendee wore a mask. The event was a success for my team; unfortunately, the pandemic was ongoing. I tallied at least 7 or 8 people infected, maybe more. Smdh. Fortunately, I didn't hear of anyone being severely ill; most of us were probably vaccinated. My symptoms consisted of a severe sore throat and nasal congestion. Tobin and Micah were only present for 1.5 hrs and were okay. Micah had it back in January.

To Have a Second Baby or Not to Have a Second Baby?

Did I want to have another child? Well, the better question was, could I have another child? Micah and I tried to conceive naturally, but nothing happened yet. Our toddler was sixteen months and a giant due to the German/Italian genes. We both had difficulties holding him, the chunky thing. Truly, we would like a second child. However, after much deliberation and reading of the statistics, another IVF journey would likely be unsuccessful for me. According to the Center for Human Reproduction, the IVF success rate for women aged forty-one was 6.7%. That was depressing to read and take in. I was lucky and grateful that my first round even took. I didn't want to retake my chances. It was emotionally risky because the disappointment would be tragic if the procedure were to fail. I am resilient with a cup-half-full mentality, but this would take a significant toll on me. The work, time, and energy I put into my body to make it baby-ready could have been a whole career. I really should have been paid for it all. Not seeing any results came with disappointment, and it was not fun. I am so lucky to be Tobin's mummy, and if he were my only child, I would be entirely content and at peace with that.

So let's talk about how some mothers just don't love being a mom, especially after being asked, *"Oh, don't you just LOVE being a mom?!"* I think we need to respect that some aren't naturally motherly in nature, and those who also love their careers. There are all types of mothers: ones that adore being a mom and nothing else, ones that, of course love their baby but it doesn't encompass their entire life, ones that would rather be hands-free and have others take care of their child, and then those who fall in-between the different levels of the spectrum, which can evolve through different life chapters. None are actually wrong or right, they just are.

I love my child and would protect him with my life. However, being a mother is not my end-all, be-all. I am more than just a mom. Some moms choose to be glued to their babies, and that sounds like a nightmare to me. I need my space, and I love my career. Also, not all moms are built the same way. Some mothers relish being stay-at-home moms and find fulfillment in this role.

On the other hand, thank the lord, baby Jesus Christ, I have a good daycare to take my toddler to four days during the work week. I think loving your baby and being a certain type of mom looks different to everyone. Although, I do find it to be sad, too, when there are mothers who live for their babies and not for themselves. This can be a slippery slope as the child grows up and becomes more independent. The mother will have difficulty adjusting to this dynamic of not being constantly needed and will have to find new meaning in their life. Also, no one likes a nagging, helicopter mom. We all need a healthy balance, and trying to have our own life will be the best example for our children. This obviously may not apply to particular circumstances, such as single mothers who don't have support or can't afford childcare. Single moms are incredible and formidable.

26. IVF is Unnatural

My girlfriends and I left our husbands for the Memorial Day weekend to a spa getaway in Leavenworth, WA, the cutest Bavarian town. The drive wasn't too bad as it was only a couple of hours away. The only problem was going through the mountain pass. My gf, who was sitting in the backseat, became carsick. Thankfully, she didn't ralph. It helped that I pulled over so she could swap seats with my gf in shotgun. We were only 20 minutes away, but I sometimes got car sick, too, so I could empathize. There were three of us, and we all had a history of being carsick, so I was glad I was driving.

Once we stepped foot into Posthotel, the aroma of pure relaxation hit our olfactory senses. Not having children present was a nice break. Children and dogs were not allowed at the spa hotel. What was also fabulous was that breakfast and lunch were included in our stay. The price tag was hefty, but it was worth every penny. The spa area was luxurious, with plenty of room to bake yourself dry in a sauna or steam yourself while lounging on slabs of marble with eucalyptus filling your lungs. Unfortunately, the hottest sauna burned my girlfriend's knees! I hoped they decreased the temperature after she notified them. The indoor pool leads to the outside through a classic arched window with a view of the mountains and river. There were a few hot tubs to soak in and cold plunges to make you tingle all over. There were lounge chairs to read in and relax, too. The rooms also had a classic Euro feel, like the hotel's. What was incredible was that each room had an all-marble bathtub that probably had not been used. The receptionist told me it took ten bloody years to finish the hotel, the same time it took to get a vaccine licensed! It was mind-boggling and deserving of much respect.

After a few hours of spa time, we got dolled up for a 5-course prix fixe dinner at Mana. The setting was so quaint. We sat in a tiny greenhouse with a heater. There were also clear igloos for smaller parties. All ingredients were from local farms, and the menu was created carefully and intentionally for the season. As we were waiting for courses to arrive, girlfriend A mentioned how she wished to have a girl, but her husband didn't want them to go through IVF because he thought it was "unnatural". She said this to girlfriend B, who went through IVF to have children. Obviously, gf A had no ill intent.

Still, the issue was that she needed to understand who her audience was and that saying certain things, even if she didn't think it was offensive, could be off-putting to others. I was also at this same table. Thus, we had two women who went through IVF directly in front of her. The more I let this comment sit, the more annoyed I became at gf A, who had a penchant for being entirely oblivious to her actions. When I met her long before this group of gfs came to be, she dismissed me. We were taking a course together, and I wanted to make friends, but she apparently had no time for that. Then, a few years later, we met again within this circle. She asked me to be her bridesmaid, which I happily accepted. I fulfilled all my duties, but then she dumped me half a year later, stating that our friendship wasn't organic enough. WTF does that even mean? Friendship takes nurturing, true intentions, and time. I was undoubtedly salty because I felt like I invested quite a bit of myself into the relationship, yet the ROI was a complete sunk cost in the long run. I was extra salty because this was the second time this chick rejected my genuine gestures of friendship. Hell hath no fury like a woman scorned.

Dispelling Myths/Trends

So, do you know how they say that breastfeeding will help you lose baby weight? Well, it didn't for me. Six months postpartum, I was a size six to eight. My chest and trunk area were still quite large for my stature. I was being hard on myself, but I was so annoyed that I could not even fit into a size small. It wasn't until Tobin began biting my boob instead of feeding, which was at about eight months, that I began to slim down due to entirely ending breastfeeding. I was probably a solid size four during the fall of 2021, and during the spring of 2022, I felt I was between a sze two to four dress size. I was pretty comfortable with that, considering I used to be a size 00 or 0. I know some women who noticed their breasts had reduced in size after having children. Mine might have been slightly larger than they were initially. Lucky Micah! Some women don't care to have sex or think it doesn't feel as good after childbirth. One person told me that she and her partner hadn't had sex since their child was born. Their child was two years old at that time. I have heard many women speak about not having any intimate moments with their partners, and they thought this was okay and that their partner should accept this. It doesn't matter if it's the woman or the man; any time a love language is not met, there will be consequences.

Once upon a time, with one of my exes (let's call him Bob), my physical love language was not being met. I had to ask for hugs and was told that I was needy because I wanted physical affection. Often, I would catch my ex after he masturbated, and I figured it out because when I got home, our bedroom blinds would be down, and I would raise them each morning. When your partner doesn't feel it is essential that your sexual needs are met, a significant strain on the relationship will be created. I was rejected time after time when I wanted to have sex with Bob. A continuum of dismissal made me feel unloved, unwanted, and undesirable. This repetition wore on me, and I fell out of love. Thus, if an individual feels their partner isn't paying attention to them, guess what? They will seek attention elsewhere or be open to it because their needs aren't being met. The moral of the story is that if you stop watering your flowers, someone else will water them for you and pluck them away. Micah entirely understands my love languages and knows what it takes to continue to sustain my love for him. He makes it his job to ensure my needs and desires are fulfilled. I am a fortunate woman to have someone who is in tune with me.

After I healed fully from delivery, it took a few months to get used to having sex, and lube was my bestie. A woman's vagina evolves, and for me, it was for the better as I became more sensitive in a good way. The second-degree tear I got from delivery made sex a bit uncomfortable at first (going slowly was my OBGYN's advice), and certain positions were not amenable, depending on the angle. In general, sex was more pleasurable; it just took time for my body to adjust. Thus, be patient with yourself.

Fertility Journey PTSD

The Kardashians were back from their hiatus. Our friends graciously allowed us to use their Hulu password, and I had been "binging" for the last few days while toddler Tobin waddled around our master bedroom and planted a greasy hand on Kourtney's face. I was enjoying this fresh new look and feel. The first episode included a brilliant opening utilizing a first-person view (FPV) drone flying in and out of each of the Kardashian dynasties. I even watched it a second time because I had to show Micah, as he had a couple of drones and created some cool videos of our travels. So I felt terrible for Scott on the show because he felt he was losing his family to Travis. Kourtney seemed so happy and gushy in love, and then the camera cut to Scott watching them interact—his face showcased how much he was dying inside. Then there were the scenes of Kourtney getting her follicles checked out by her fertility doctor.

The doc explained how one of the follicles looked expired, and then when he looked at the other ovary, he saw one big follicle, which hopefully housed the prized golden egg. I had a visceral reaction while watching Kourtney and Travis pray that her egg retrieval would be successful. I recalled the feelings of anxiousness at each ultrasound appointment and the nervous clasping of my hands while my follicles were measured. It was unnerving not to be in control of how my body reacted to the hormones and how well the eggs would develop. These scenes triggered me, and I could empathize entirely with Kourtney. I felt bad for her struggle, and to watch her speak about how her egg retrieval was not successful was quite heartbreaking. This was what I worried about if I tried IVF again. I was unsure how many disappointments I could take and if I wanted to risk my mental stability. I did feel that I should see an acupuncturist again.

Toxicity

Mothers endure way too much, especially when they are already exhausted and drained from taking care of their babies. Thus, clearing your life of those who are toxic and do not fully support you need to be exiled from your village. The infinite number of stories about in-laws who lacked respect and criticized the new mothers was abhorrent. I needed to stop reading these rants because the negative energy spread through these posts. At the very least, I tried to respond to some with supportive suggestions and with empathy or sympathy.

The latest story I read was of a woman who believed she would get pregnant straight away (like me) and didn't. When she finally became pregnant, she miscarried and went through numerous miscarriages afterward. When they received their fertility test results, she looked good on paper, while her husband had wonky sperm. He refused to have further genetic tests done. The MIL kept asking insane questions like, "What did you eat? What were you doing? How did you kill your baby this time?" What made me cringe even more about this story was that the MIL was Vietnamese. The stereotypes continued to be perpetuated on their own accord. This reminded me of Ali Wong's comic routine, in which she spoke about miscarriages, and people asked her, "What did you do?" Blaming women for the loss of their unborn children was not only undeniably wrong but completely inaccurate.

The zygote won't survive if the protein sequences, aka DNA, are not correctly formed. Cell death will occur because everything shuts down if things aren't replicating normally. This is how the zygote ensures its success. If the mechanics aren't working, then self-termination is inevitable. Essentially, this is a prime example of survival of the fittest in the womb. Women don't cause miscarriages; DNA errors do. Errors in DNA can be due to a variety of factors. One thing we can't do is put full blame on the woman because the sperm also has a 50% role in the formation of the embryo. This is a joint effort, and pointing fingers helps no one.

The lack of support and understanding for mothers who miscarry was frustrating and lonely. Small comments like, "Oh, you can just try again" or "You'll get over it someday" are highly unhelpful. I felt like I wasn't being a comforting friend to my gf when she had a miscarriage many years ago when I wasn't on my fertility journey. I had no clue about what she was going through at all, and I couldn't understand why she was still so sad about it, even when her healthy son was about to turn five. She told me that she still thought about her first pregnancy and what could have been. A loss was still a loss, and I should have been more sympathetic towards her.

I want every mother to know they control who they allow in their precious circle. If there is even an iota of disrespect or support, please distance yourself, especially if they are your family. Familial ties do not excuse rudeness or offensive behaviors. Boundaries are essential for your mental well-being.

27. Partnership

I was lucky and grateful for my husband. Yes, that sounded like a super cheesy IG caption, but it was true. Micah and I were on the same page, and our values aligned. And, if, for some reason, we were not in agreement, the communication line was always opened and transparent. Many women expected their partners to read their minds, which was so juvenile. Let's be clear: nobody can read your mind, and you shouldn't put others through petty tests, which will always end in disappointment. I was rarely disappointed because I always told Micah what was happening in my head. Many asked me if Micah had helped with the baby, and I told all of them that he had entirely! The duties were pretty 50/50 between us. I also went on girls' trips at least once a year, so he took care of the baby more than I did. I think there were a few reasons for this dynamic and absolute responsibility. Firstly, Micah wanted a baby before me. This yearning to be a father was key to having a present and active one. Secondly, my job was the most important one to keep, as I earned more money. This was actually a phenomenon I observed in my circle of friends, many of whom were the breadwinners and mothers. Seeing intelligent women of color (WOC) leaders in their fields was inspirational.

Anyhow, back to how amazing Micah was. Not only was he a trophy husband, but he also knew my love languages. This was key to our successful marriage. Everyone should learn to identify what they value in relationships. My top three love languages were physical touch, quality time, and acts of service. If your top three are not met most of the time, then problems will arise. That was what occurred in my first marriage, and we divorced. I felt like divorce was underrated. Staying in a loveless relationship would eventually kill you inside. I found it amazing that many thought they had to sacrifice everything for their marriage, thus electing to become martyrs. This was the recipe for resentment.

Online, there were numerous posts seeking advice on staying in the marriage for the sake of the kids. Those who grew up in households with parents who hated each other and fought non-stop wished their parents had filed for divorce. The negative energy and hostility became palpable, and the kids saw and heard everything. The example set for these children was a horrible one, which carried into adulthood and their relationships.

One partnership trend I noticed was where households were a strict 50/50 split, even if one partner made significantly more than the other. When Micah and I first began dating and living together, everything was split down the middle. This was entirely fair because, even though I was a full-time student, I did not expect him to cover all of my living costs; as an independent adult woman, I should bring something to the table. We had an argument (probably right before I was about to get my period) about expenses and how I thought he should pay a bit more on his end because he was my boyfriend, but reflecting back, that didn't make sense. I was separated from my rich ex-husband and no longer living in Madison Park (a very nice area in Seattle) so maybe I felt entitled to anything. Perhaps I just wanted to be treated out a little more. Micah did try to accommodate me in certain ways by paying fully for our date nights, which was sweet and considerate, especially since I was living off my student loans, training grants, and scholarships. Truly, the whole sentiment of the man paying for everything continues the patriarchal paradigm that society still embraces fully. These archaic practices have naturally evolved since women have full-time careers and are having children at much later ages. Plus, more women now hold better and higher-paying jobs than their male counterparts. After about three years of living together, Micah began to make more money, and we moved into a townhouse together. I had to sacrifice my cute, zippy Scion TC and sell it to pay off Micah's Prius payments, thereby balancing his income-to-debt ratio. Essentially, we were banking on his income to help us purchase our first home together, but we contributed differently. I would be damned if my name was not on the deed, and Micah had no qualms with me owning half of the house. By the time we moved in, Micah was paying the mortgage entirely, as my funds had run out about a year before I graduated from my PhD program. Thus, he invested in our future together and understood that if he didn't help support me during my schooling, we wouldn't succeed together as partners. Now, I make more than him, and a 50/50 split would be unfair. I am happy to pay more for our bills because it doesn't make sense to bleed him dry. He needs his own financial security.

In general, when it comes to finances, no one should expect anything except to go dutch for a while in a new relationship. However, in certain circumstances, one partner may have to pay more for the living expenses. Again, this should never be expected, and multiple conversations must occur. As modern-day women, we should never count on anyone to pay for our expenses, and we certainly can't count on others to help us survive. If something doesn't pan out, we must always have multiple backup plans (A, B, C) in place. Financial independence is essential - it's survival 101.

Moving on to other problematic situations, I would like to take the time to reflect on stories I have heard about wives who caught their husbands cheating on them with prostitutes, then blaming it on sex addiction, then threatening to harm themselves, and promising they will change. Why do women take the vows "in sickness and in health" so bloody seriously? I mean, way more seriously than men do? Is it all of the Disney princess movies they watched during childhood, the super saccharine rom coms, K dramas, or the cheesiness of Love Actually? These husbands probably passed on sexually transmitted infections to their wives. It truly doesn't matter how good a father they are because he was a terrible husband and partner to his wife. Children see everything. They internalize it and unconsciously mirror the experiences they had while growing up. Daughters need to witness good, solid examples of self-respect, self-dignity, self-confidence, and high self-esteem. They will grow up thinking the way their father behaves is acceptable. Imploring to end one's life to be forgiven is manipulation at its finest. Rehabilitation and counseling may help, but the damage has already been done. Normally, addicts in general will relapse repeatedly, and it is not a pretty sight. People with an addiction say they will change over and over again, and they do want to, but the addiction is too strong to overcome. It's the worst rollercoaster ride to endure.

I want to be extremely clear about this point—marriage vows do not mean we should never divorce our husbands. Ladies, we are not chained to our words on our wedding day. Life is unpredictable, and people can break their promises. Women need to respect and love themselves first. We are the priority in our lives, and we should always put ourselves first before anyone else. We are ultimately in charge of our fate and manifesting our destiny. No one else is here to create the world we want to live in. We build it and are in control of it. No one is here to make us happy; we need to produce that happiness for ourselves. We deserve to be cherished, respected, and loved *all the time*, not sometimes.

28. Make It Easy For Yourself

Many mothers believe they must give their babies every ounce of themselves. If they do"t, they will feel ultimate guilt. I have observed that if mum isn't happy, no one is. If you can make your life easier, take all those opportunities. One prime example was sleep time. We had never co-slept with Tobin. He always went down in his crib. Parents need time to unwind and relax; we can't do that with a child sleeping by our side. According to the Australian Parenting Website, co-sleeping was associated with an increased risk of sudden unexpected death in infancy (SUDI). In certain circumstances, parents felt the need for co-sleeping, and this website provided advice on the safest ways to do so.

The more babies can sleep independently, the more time parents have available. We began sleep training at seven months, which was successful within the first week. We utilized the Ferber method and adjusted it to what we could tolerate regarding the crying. I would sing to him, rock him for a few songs, and then put him down to sleep. Initially, I let him cry for about ten to twelve minutes, then I went back in and comforted him a bit while he was still in his crib, then left again. This repeated about three times, and then he got used to self-soothing. The pattern eventually worked, and the baby learned to fall asleep independently. Our toddler slept through the night every night for at least eleven hours. He slept with a pacifier, which probably contributed significantly to his ability to sleep independently and self-soothe. During the day, he took two naps, but when he was at daycare, which began at eighteen months, they only did one nap lasting one to two hours.

Trusting strangers to take care of your baby can be unnerving. I tried not to look at too many horror news stories about babies being harmed by their hired caretakers, but I wanted to inform myself as much as possible to prevent future danger. We only had one option for daycare, so we chose it. The reviews seemed fine, and everything looked normal when we took a tour. Micah didn't like how the toddlers and teachers wore outdoor shoes in the room. I trained this man pretty well by having shoes off at home.

During the pandemic, childcare services were limited due to staffing shortages. This same daycare had to close its infant program (for children under seventeen months) because they could not hire enough staff. Recently, I heard on the news that another daycare gave parents seventeen days' notice that they were closing due to leasing issues. Parents were working from home (WFH)) and having to watch their child simultaneously. All of these challenges were truly unprecedented and weren't getting better. With great resignation, I was perplexed about what people did if they weren't working and how they paid their bills.

I recall hearing about a mother who felt completely inadequate. She had a toddler and seriously felt that her husband and child would be fine if she had left. This mom was completely burnt out in Toddlerville with endless tantrums, where the baby preferred daddy most of the time. She felt rejected by her own biological child and was pained by this. She also mourned the life she used to have pre-baby. Apparently, this husband mentioned that he never wanted to travel without their child, so there would never be a moment when it would just be the two of them alone. This wife no longer felt like a priority. The thought of bringing a kicking and screaming child on a plane gave her an incredible amount of anxiety. She has also considered leaving the family on several occasions. This poor woman was feeling entirely inadequate. Hopefully, this was just a toddler stage, but it must be rough. I heard mothers speak about mourning their lives pre-baby and fantasizing about the days of their liberty. Adjusting to the needs/priorities of your little one can be difficult, and if your partner is not willing to take vacations without them, that is a tough pill to swallow. I thought she needed to discuss this further with him and decide to have just couples time. Partners occasionally need some breathing room from their parental duties because they still need to spend time courting each other. It is similar to a muscle; you lose it or become weak if you don't use it. Quality time together and a showcase of love and affection are pertinent for relationship survival. This also acts as an excellent example of healthy partnerships for their children. Feelings of wanting to escape are very dangerous. Possibly her husband was not doing enough to make her feel loved, wanted, and supported. This would be much to unpack with a

129

therapist. This poor woman sounded defeated. Her cup was completely empty, and no one was seeing this.

<u>Winning at Work Again</u>

I got back from a face-to-face team meeting in Milwaukee. Why there, you ask? Great question. My director wanted us to meet somewhere central. I would have preferred a spot on the West Coast. Our medical affairs team had not seen each other in person for two years, so this was a big deal. There were four new people on my US team whom I had never met in person, only virtually. The energy of personalities colliding in the flesh is incomparable to a virtual meeting. Lively banter and hearty laughter are energizing for this ambivert.

My manager was on medical leave for the last month and a half, and I was entrusted with being the interim manager. It was a terrific development opportunity for me, and it was great to be trusted and recognized by my directors. I was asked to meet with my manager and two directors on our last day in Milwaukee. All four of us walked out of the meeting room and down the hall. One of our colleagues made a funny, incoherent noise as we marched past, probably wondering what the procession was all about. We sat down in the lounge area, which was currently vacant because it was 8:30 a.m. They all took turns thanking me for stepping in and spoke highly of me.

I felt so appreciated and didn't think my career could provide a great sense of fulfillment. The cherry on top was that I was getting a raise. It was evident that my higher-ups wanted to retain me. Because I exceeded my 2021-22 fiscal year objectives, I also received an additional bonus. While I was a student, I firmly thought that work would be so dreary and boring. I loved learning and the liberties that came with it, but little did I realize that you truly can be content with your daily job and earn a terrific salary. These amazing things did not just fall into my lap; I created and manifested my destiny. For example, the first time I asked for a raise, I had only been in my job for two years. However, I knew my worth and that there was room for negotiation. I never turned down a new challenge or project and made myself available to my manager as much as possible for delegated tasks. These opportunities have created visibility within my role, which is essential to be seen as a valuable player. The moral of the story is that you must ask and be open to opportunities. Status quo won't get you anywhere.

Many women do not deem themselves valuable team members, nor do they realize that they bring a rare expertise. Ladies, you are a diamond worth the company's highest amount. If the salary goes as high as $150K, you'd better bloody demand that amount. Women continue to earn less than their male counterparts. Thus, you should not settle for just what you think you need. Know your worth! When a company offers you a job, they want YOU. Therefore, it would be entirely appropriate for you to come in and negotiate your salary. One of my friends, who has been a recruiter for a long time, expects negotiations to occur. Mind you, she is in tech, and each industry may differ, but you should still ask for the highest salary you can get with your position.

The Musks

So I hate to bring up Elon again, but he secretly had another child via surrogacy with Grimes. Their daughter was born in December 2021. Then, it was recently revealed that he had a set of twins with one of his top executives in the same year. And now there are rumors that Amber Heard's child could be Elon's via surrogacy! Wait, it gets even better! Elon's father just had a child with his own bloody stepdaughter, who is forty-one years his junior (he's seventy-six, she's thirty-five). And, get this!! It is his second child with her! You can't make this shizzz up. Seriously! His exact words: "The only thing we are on earth for is to reproduce." Like father, like son. Wow. The Musk dynasty is no joke, and I am sure King Elon's DNA will survive an apocalypse.

It is interesting to see how couples evolve. Some want children or to adopt them, only to realize one day that they don't. Others are so adamant about not having any, and then they are surprised when they are expecting. There are women who suddenly one day feel a sense of urgency to have one. It must be their biological clock and a surge of hormones. How funny to completely change your ideation after so many years. These moms who have a change of heart tend to want more than just one child, too, and then have to persuade their partners to have more. Basically, if one parent doesn't want more children, then the answer should be no, period. If the tables were turned and a man was forcing a woman to have a child, we would all scream bloody murder!!

Astonishingly, certain folks think bringing another child into this world is okay when only one parent is up for it. It's manipulative to even think that a parent who is not on board would eventually come around. The moral of the story is that if your partner doesn't want more kids, this should not be dismissed based on your hormonal clock, AND you shouldn't have more. Apparently, getting a puppy is a good solution for some.

29. AAP Recommendations For Breastfeeding

On June 27, 2022, the American Academy of Pediatrics (AAP) published an article titled *Technical Report: Breastfeeding and the Use of Human Milk*. It called for more support for breastfeeding mothers. The article identified stigma, lack of support, and workplace barriers as obstacles that hindered continued breastfeeding.

This first statement was helpful as it pointed out significant challenges when it came to breastfeeding. Essentially, society as a whole does not do enough to support mothers who choose to breastfeed.

The AAP recommended exclusive breastfeeding of infants for the first six months of life before introducing nutritious complementary foods while encouraging social and systemic changes to support mothers who choose to breastfeed. I thought this recommendation of exclusive breastfeeding for six months was quite insensitive. Like, how feasible was this, especially for working mothers, and could this actually be implemented? The answer is, for mothers in the US, where there is no universal paid parental leave, it's unrealistic and a fantasy. According to Wikipedia, the USA, Papua New Guinea, and a few island countries in the Pacific Ocean are the only countries in the United Nations that do not require employers to provide paid time off for new parents. One mother told me that she gave birth to her child and had to get back to work within three weeks because she didn't have any more paid time off (PTO) to use, and she needed to keep her job. This was one of the saddest things I ever heard about being a new mother. So AAP expected moms to continue to breastfeed their child when they have to go to work for at least 8 hours a day, where we would essentially have to pump every couple hours. How do we find the time to go to a private, quiet spot and pump in peace? What if there wasn't a peaceful, private place for moms to pump? What if our job was customer or patient-facing? Would our boss be okay with us having all these "breaks" during working hours for six months? The biggest issue with this statement was, what if the mother couldn't make enough milk? Then we'd feel guilty because AAP said we should be doing this. Not only that, but we take a course on breastfeeding where the nurse tells us that "breast is best" and never mentions that we could have issues with our baby latching on or that we may not make enough milk and would have to supplement with formula. The stories I have read about mothers so deep in desperation to get their breasts to produce an ample amount of liquid gold are disheartening.

In the July 2022 issue of Pediatrics, the AAP outlined its recommendations and evidence of significant health benefits to infants and mothers who chose to breastfeed their infant to age **two** and beyond. Ok, are you effin' kidding me right now? How the hell would working mothers (the ones who can actually produce enough milk) do this? If you worked at an Amazon warehouse, you wouldn't be allowed to leave your demanding job of fulfilling infinite orders to pump and store your milk. If you worked as a barista at Starbucks, would your manager let you leave the espresso machine for 15-20 minutes every few hours to pump? What about those who worked at a hospital or a restaurant where you serviced people? There was no way. I had to stop breastfeeding my son at eight months because he began to bite my nipples, and I wanted to keep them intact thank you very much. He even found it funny when I told him "no." I did my best, but I didn't even get up to a full year of breastfeeding, AND I had to supplement with formula because I wasn't making enough for him to get full. He was always a big eater.

The other important part was that mothers needed space and time to recharge. The expectation of being a full-time food producer, caretaker, cleaner, cook, career woman, and more was unrealistic and put enormous pressure on moms. It was just way too much!

"Human milk is all a baby needs for the first six months of life," said Joan Younger Meek, MD, MS, RD, FAAP, FABM, IBCLC, lead author of the reports written by the AAP section on breastfeeding. "Breast milk is unique in its nutrients and protective effects, and really quite remarkable when you look at what it does for a child's developing immune system. Not everyone can breastfeed or continue breastfeeding for as long as desired for various reasons, including workplace barriers.

134

Families deserve nonjudgmental support, information and help to guide them in feeding their infant."

Research showed that breastfeeding decreased rates of lower respiratory tract infections, severe diarrhea, ear infections, and obesity. It was also associated with a lower risk of sudden infant death syndrome and other protective effects. Again, that was good to know, but not doable in America. Plus, my pediatrician told me to start introducing mushed solids at four months, which worked out well for my baby. He became a solid food eater much quicker than we expected and loved the variety.

The AAP recommended:

Exclusive breastfeeding for the first six months. There was no need to introduce infant formula or other sources of nutrition for most infants. Beyond six months, breastfeeding should be maintained along with nutritious complementary foods.

Birth hospitals or centers implement maternity care practices that improve breastfeeding initiation, duration, and exclusivity.

Breastfeeding beyond one year and up to 2 years. Long-term breastfeeding was especially beneficial for the mother and was associated with protection against diabetes, high blood pressure, and cancers of the breast and ovaries.

Mothers who chose to breastfeed beyond the first year needed support from their medical care providers as well as protections against workplace barriers.

Policies that protected breastfeeding, including universal paid maternity leave, the right of a woman to breastfeed in public, insurance coverage for lactation support and breast pumps, on-site child care, universal workplace break time with a clean, private location for expressing milk, the right to feed expressed milk, and the right to breastfeed in child care centers and lactation rooms in schools to supporting families in sustaining breastfeeding.

Again, more fantasies that would never come true, especially the last bullet point about universal workplace break time with a clean, private space for expressing milk. This was America, where capitalism kept the nation's heart, aka bank, pumping. There was too much money to be made and too many employees to underpay. I appreciated what AAP recommended but wanted to know what they did to make this a reality. Did they have lobbyists advocating for their recommendations? Or were these all just words? In a nation where healthcare is not universal, the future for policy change on breastfeeding is abysmal.

"The AAP views breastfeeding as a public health imperative and also as an equity issue," said Lawrence Noble, MD, FAAP, FABM, IBCLC, co-author of the policy statement and technical report, which detailed the evidence supporting human milk feeding. "Pediatricians and other medical professionals can help mothers meet their intended goals for breastfeeding and provide care that is inclusive, equitable, and culturally sensitive."

According to the 2018 National Immunization Survey (NIS) of the Centers for Disease Control and Prevention, White, Hispanic, Latino, and Asian families initiated breastfeeding at higher rates than the Black population in the United States,. Similar disparities were also seen among low-income mothers who participated in the Special Supplemental Nutrition Program for Women, Infants, and Children (WIC), women younger than twenty, and those with a high school education or less. The policy statement called for addressing implicit bias, structural bias, and structural racism to eliminate disparities in breastfeeding and improve the health and well-being of all children and families.

AAP addressed the disparity in Black populations, but what were pediatricians doing about these issues? What was America doing about this steep imbalance? You were out of luck unless you worked for a corporation with socialistic roots. America loves money, and capitalism rules the nation. What the leaders of this nation do not understand is that supporting parents both monetarily and emotionally creates healthier and more successful societies because future generations will have a higher chance of thriving. However, there is also a vicious poverty cycle where those on the lower socioeconomic level stay there because there is a lack of proper policies that address and remedy issues on equity, access, resources, housing, fair wages, mental health, etc. The list goes on. You can tell someone that they should breastfeed because it's good for their baby, but if they can't because they have to go back to work right after giving birth, then these recommendations are pretty useless. Essentially, you can't get to step number five without climbing the first four steps.

The policy also noted that children of gender-diverse parents may have less access to human milk because of both social and biological constraints. When working with gender-diverse families, AAP suggested asking families what terms they use and that the term "chestfeeding" may be more accurate and inclusive as it concerns lactation and physiology in gender-diverse families.

"Breastfeeding can be challenging for new parents, and support from their families, doctors, and workplaces is essential," Dr. Meek said. "The health benefits are vast and can be viewed as a long-term investment not only in a child's development but to public health as a whole."

I'm glad they included the DEI statement with super PC labels. Chestfeeding was even a new one for me. As for the second statement, again, there were many words, but where was the action? Being able to breastfeed your baby for an extended period of time is basically a privilege in America. The other part involved very expensive lactation consults. I have insurance and still have to pay for some of my appointments. Thus, there is a lack of accessibility. When you are a first-time mother, learning how to breastfeed and getting your baby to learn can be very difficult. The nuances involved within this subject are complex, and the foundation lies within universal, paid parental leave.

30. Cultural Differences

My first long-term relationship began when I was sixteen with an Asian male. Let's call him Archie. Before that, I also had other Asian "boyfriends," which only lasted a few months. This first serious relationship was dysfunctional in that open communication was lacking. Archie was quite secretive for no apparent reason. He seemed mysterious to me; he even had a friendship with a younger girl who seemed suspicious. I didn't even know if he graduated high school. He was at least a year or two older than me. Ya, he was even secretive about his age so I didn't know the year he was born. The summer I graduated from high school in 1999, Archie seemed distant, and I was immaturely testing him to see if he would change his ways and be a better boyfriend to me. One of these tests was to see if he would ask me to dance during my graduation celebration. (By the way, Canadians call prom grad.) A slow song came on, and Archie just sat there, so I went over to my white guy friend, Zach, and asked him to dance instead. This shocked Archie a bit, but I didn't care. I was done with his complacency.

Interestingly enough, I developed feelings for Zach. He was the complete opposite of Archie—tall, white, blue-green eyes, way more communicative, and paid attention to me. For me, this was the turning point where I pretty much vowed not to date Asian guys again. Archie's behaviors within our relationship completely turned me off, and I never wanted to return to that. Unfortunately, I made a broad generalization about all Asian men due to him. However, my physical attraction to white men increased when I turned eighteen. Perhaps these two turning points were interrelated.

Since then, I had four serious relationships with white men, including Micah. Two of them were hilarious Jewish men. Mind you, dealing with the Jewish women (ie. mom, sister, grandma) in their lives was like being in a lion's den but I do cherish the times I was treated like family. I had to put up with a lot of disrespect being a shiksa (non-Jewish girl), but perhaps I paved the way for future partners who also were not Jewish. When it came to dating white men, there were notable cultural differences compared to dating Asian men who came from traditional Asian households (the ones who are Americanized are a bit of a different story).

First, let's talk about money. My single girlfriends often commented how going on a date with a white man was pretty different from Asian ones. I could attest to this. Most white men expect women to go dutch during the first few dates, i.e., a fifty-fifty split. Most Asian men usually pay for the whole bill, and the first date is typically a nice dinner, whereas the first date with some white guys consists of just coffee or tea. I mean, dating can be costly for a bachelor. Thus, I suppose having a simple, low-risk encounter is easier on the pocket, and you can gauge from there whether a second date is worthwhile. My gfs also mentioned that Asian guys seem to be more considerate of where you are located and will either pick you up for a date or meet you close to where you live. The white guys will offer to meet up halfway at best. Unfortunately, these mannerisms painted a lazy first impression.

So, let's fast forward to being in a committed partnership with a white guy. I got used to splitting everything fifty-fifty as this was now the norm - all bills, rent, etc, were distributed equally. There was even an Excel sheet of all the combined expenses and who paid for what, so everything was fair and square. Let's be fair, though; sometimes, my white man would pay for the entire dinner bill on fancy date nights. So, where did these practices originate from, and why did the more traditional Asian men have less of a problem taking care of most of the finances? This was definitely a cultural aspect where, in Asian families, the patriarchy was still very strong, and some Asian women (even modern ones) had a sense of entitlement and/or expectation that their men would take care of them. There was undoubtedly a set of expectations in Asian culture that were not present in white households, and this was where problems arose once the interracial couple got married and had children. However, I might add that there are Asian households where the matriarch is the breadwinner, which was my case where my mother was well-educated.

Let's look at one example scenario I felt was commonplace. One fine summer back in 2012, Micah and I were invited to a wedding, and we discussed how much to give the bride and groom. Asians are pretty generous and will gift the newlyweds at least $200. Plus, I believe the etiquette should be at least $75-$100 per person because I don't want to just pay for the meal; I want to contribute a bit more to help support the couple. Micah thought this amount was ludicrous and felt $100 max was going above and beyond. In fact, for our own wedding, a family member (non-Asian) only gave $50 total for their family of *FOUR* (each of the adult meals was at least $50 and the kids were $25 a pop). I don't think they were struggling at the time but what do I know. So, was this cheap, or was it a cultural thing? I believe the answer is both because another family member (non-Asian) didn't give us anything and there were three of them.

In my experience, Micah had never attended weddings with his parents and thus never experienced any of the practices or understood the nuances. Plus, there were times when his family was not doing well, so there was the poor card, too. This situation was entirely understandable; he was ignorant of proper wedding gift etiquette. I couldn't blame him for it. Thus, I had to come in and educate him. It was interesting because Micah would be frugal on some things, and I would be frugal on others. For example, he would rather pay an extra $10 bucks on garbage day to pick up our extra bag that won't fit in the bin, while I would rather wait until next week when our garbage was less full. I mean, that's ten whole bucks wasted! Just wait another bloody week!

I had this Asian guy friend, Leo, who was in an interesting predicament with one of his previous, quite traditional, Asian girlfriends. Leo was brought up in a very non-traditional household. Culturally speaking, he was pretty much white. This new gf, Tiffany, got irritated with him when they went out on dates, and he could not understand the issue until they finally sat down and had a conversation. She was miffed because she didn't care for going dutch on their dates. Essentially, she expected him to pay for all of their outings. Tiffany's love language was acts of service. If she invited him to dinner, she would take care of everything. After overcoming this incident, things went well. Leo didn't mind taking care of the bill more often than before, and everything seemed dandy. After a few weeks, Tiffany appeared irritated again, and Leo had to decipher the issue. They had been a few months into their serious relationship, but

Tiffany was still unsatisfied with their arrangement. Her besties had bfs who paid for everything and even let them go shopping with their credit cards. She had the audacity to exclaim that what was hers was hers and what was his was hers.

Now hold your darn tootin' horses, Tiffany! This behavior was distasteful, especially for an adult millennial woman. We have evolved from archaic times when men took care of everything; in fact, partnerships have evolved because of feminism and the state of the economy. Many households need both partners to make a decent living, even to afford a condo or townhouse, as the housing market has skyrocketed and salaries have not followed suit. Thus, expecting your bf of a few months to take care of all the expenses you both incurred, not to mention claiming his hard-earned money as your own, was so bloody basic and unrealistic. I mean, you would be better off being a sugar baby. This relationship didn't last very long, and Tiffany was devastated that Leo had dumped her. Just because you're cute doesn't mean you get to have all his money.

Going back to my mother being the breadwinner and the fact that I am not from a super traditional household… I don't scoff at going dutch at the beginning of a relationship. In fact, I don't expect to be anybody's dependent nor would I choose to be - life can be unfair, cruel, and unpredictable. A woman should be prepared for any situation that may arise. I have read stories where women wanted to leave but had no savings or control of the finances and was inextricably bound to their husband. This was a precarious and dangerous situation to be in. I never wanted to create that world for myself nor my children.

Another substantial cultural difference was the acceptance of toxic behaviors and dysfunctional family environments. Some of the norms in many Asian families are being brutally honest, making crude comments, always respecting your elders no matter how horrible they are to you, obeying your parents at all times, being taken for granted, and always seeing the negative side of every situation. This may be entirely unfamiliar to white partners who never fully comprehend these dynamics. Their first reaction would be shock because they would never put up with this if they were treated in this manner. Then, after more time with observations/encounters, usually, your non-Asian partner would say something and become livid because they can no longer stand the ill-treatment. And, if boundaries were not set correctly or toxic behaviors didn't change, resentment and hatred would come in. It's never a good time when your husband can't stand your family.

I heard about how someone's mother kept criticizing her attire and told her how she looked like a hobo. The mother would ask why her daughter didn't dress nicely, would be disappointed because she didn't converse with her enough during dinner (mind you, she had two little ones to look after), and criticized her for not smiling more often because it was unattractive not to look happy. Her husband was Asian. He tried to minimize the damage with conversational distractions. If you have two Asians who are used to this, then boundaries may have never been established. Sometimes, you need an outsider to remind you that you don't deserve to be treated like this by anyone, including the people who brought you into this world. Disrespect from anyone is never acceptable.

The older generations value perfect impressions, and we modern women understand that is fake BS. We would rather be true to ourselves than save face or be something we are not. We value genuine people and don't see the necessity of fancy jewelry and designer handbags. Of course, we still buy these things, but we are not beholden to our material possessions. The point was that Asian parents and grandparents pick at every little thing and won't stop. It's demeaning and degrading. If they don't change, you must remove yourself.

31. New Acupuncturist

I was reluctant to use a new acupuncture practitioner because my previous one was so good! I reunited with Tate as she had an opening, so I decided to see her one last time before switching to someone in my area. She had been on maternity leave for the entire pandemic and just returned a few months ago. Tate was elated to see photos of my toddler and could not believe he was 18 months old. I told her that my soon-to-be acupuncturist was a newbie and would be supervised, which was a bit concerning, but she thought it would probably be okay. I was glad I got one last session with the practitioner I connected with, and she was the one I felt helped me greatly during my journey. I am forever grateful for her assistance and expertise.

A few weeks after this appointment, I was able to get in a bit sooner with the newbie, Reagan. Her supervisor, Dr. Y, who owned the practice, was an Asian-American woman, which I appreciated. I went through my medical history with Reagan, who furiously took notes. They checked my tongue and pulse before poking me with tiny, sharp, metal objects. Reagan was the stereotypical yoga instructor with luscious wavy brown hair, a fit, calm aura, and a sparkle in her green/amber eyes. She wouldn't stop saying how "beautiful" everything was. Like, "Wow, what a beautiful story," or "That's super beautiful," or "Thank you for sharing your beautiful journey."

I am not making fun of her. I liked her a lot. It was just a bit comedic to me, the very in-touch hippie archetype she represented. It was also kind of a Pacific Northwest Yogi masterlike thing. After I lay down, it took a while to get back to me because Reagan and Dr. Y were probably deliberating on where to poke me. Finally, they came in, and both of them placed needles on me in tandem. Most of the pokes hurt and ached because I hadn't been in a while and because they poked a bit too deeply in certain spots. I tried hard to endure and accept the pain but got them to dial back a bit in some areas.

The worst was the point in the center of the sole of my foot. I have plantar fasciitis (super flat feet), which causes some discomfort and muscle soreness in my calves. Reagan only did my left foot because I did not want to feel the same thing on my right foot. I had needles near my neck and shoulder area, my arms and hands, my abdomen, legs, and feet. It was quite a spectacle; This was the most needle-filled experience ever. I appreciated the thoroughness, actually. I felt that previous acupuncturists were more focused on the fertility aspect, where this felt like a whole-body experience. I guess that was expected since my insurance didn't cover fertility but covered body pain, and I had quite a bit of discomfort within my body that needed to be taken care of. The part that gave me much discomfort was the back of my hips, which was probably a residual aftereffect of delivery.

After my session, we discussed why my fertility specialist had recommended proceeding with IVF since Reagan felt my hormone levels were adequate and I was healthy overall. This was the first time a practitioner told me I shouldn't have gone through IVF. Obviously, it was too late for that, but she indicated she would not have recommended IVF for me. I told her we felt a sense of urgency because I was 38 then. Reagan understood that sentiment, but I thought she wasn't entirely convinced of my fertility specialist's decision or at least the authorization of it. I mean, of course, the fertility clinics wanted my money; it was a business, after all, but perhaps Reagan had a point. However, even if I had chosen a different path, nothing was guaranteed, and doing IVF was meant to be at that time. They suggested I redo my hormone panel, so I made an appointment to have my blood drawn at my doctor's office.

The doctor tested AMH, FSH, LH, and estrogen levels. At first, my doctor's office didn't include AMH, so I had to request it. Patients need to be educated and advocate for themselves. Yes, we should trust our practitioners and have confidence in them, but they can't remember everything (especially when it comes to specialized medicine) and are human. As soon as I received my results, I forwarded them to Dr. Y, my first contact with the acupuncture office. I was shocked to see the result for my AMH level, which was 0.798. Right before I did my IVF cycle, my AMH was at 0.5, and that had decreased when I first had it tested before I did those rounds of IUIs (it was 0.7 initially). I researched if AMH levels could increase, and miraculously, they can. My excitement fluttered that morning, and I wondered if I should do another round of IVF to try to produce multiple viable embryos. I would be elated if I had more than one, given my age and previous experience.

On my third visit, Reagan was out of the office. Dr. Y poked me that day. She reviewed my results and said they were in the normal range. Their regular regimen would be to try Chinese herbs naturally for at least three months. Since there would be a few weeks of gap in my acupuncture due to scheduling conflicts, Dr. Y said it would be best to discuss this further when we get on a more regular schedule.

It was now the beginning of October, and I could get on a weekly acupuncture schedule, which cost me $90 per session. This increased by $20 since I did it back in 2019. I wondered if I should go every other week, but I had to have my chi reset and increase my blood circulation. Thus, I stuck with my next six weeks of booked appointments. It had been at least a month since I saw Reagan. She asked some questions to remind herself of my situation, and I did have some updates. My cycles were usually every 27-28 days and rarely deviated from the schedule. I expected to have my period on Friday, but I began my period on day 25. On day 24, I felt intense cramping, which was abnormal for me, and I saw some discharge with a light pink hue. I wasn't sure what was going on. Reagan thought this was peculiar as well. I mentioned that I was in Keystone, Colorado, at a conference last week, and the altitude was 10,804 feet above sea level. I wondered if this could have affected my regular cycle. She thought it was rare but possible since high elevations caused fluctuations in hormone levels. By the way, Seattle is literally at sea level. Thus, this could have been a thing since I was not used to such high altitudes. Anyhow, Reagan went a bit crazy with the needles this round. She forgot to take one out at the end of my appointment but to be fair, it was in my hip with my underwear covering it.

One new regimen I acquired from Reagan was seed cycling. It involved making these power seed balls that contained peanut butter and ground up seeds. Seed cycling is the rotation of specific seeds between the two main menstrual cycle phases - the follicular and luteal phases (theemilymorrow.com). The primary outcome was to help regulate and

145

balance estrogen and progesterone within our bodies. Apparently, this could help with PMS, acne, weight gain, mood swings, libido, fatigue, healing, and other fertility issues. During the follicular phase (days 1-13), you increase your flax and pumpkin seed intake; for the luteal phase (days 14-28), it's sesame and sunflower seeds. I had delegated Micah to make me my seed balls.

The blogger, Emily Morrow, indicated that it might take three to four months to notice any significant changes. Still, she noted feeling different in the first thirty days, where she had no symptoms during her period, i.e., bloating, cramps, fatigue, or headache. Eating one of these balls every morning was filling, and I had one with my tea. I tried to monitor any significant changes. Dr. Y even gave me tea to drink, which was a bitter, ground-up concoction I needed to take twice daily. I filled a large shot glass with hot water, put four scoops of ground dust, and stirred with a chopstick. While drinking this shot, I closed my nasal passages and chased it down with water and Chex cereal. It was $23 a week for a bottle of bitter dust. I wondered how sustainable this was for me.

After over a month of the regimen, I had to stop cold turkey. My body is very sensitive to any substance, natural or synthetic. Too much of anything can be bad, and the tea and ground-up seed balls made me feel weird and unwell. It worked, but it was not beneficial. If it doesn't make you feel well don't continue. Now, I need to deal with the bag of unground flaxseeds, sunflower seeds, and half a bottle of awful Chinese herbs.

32. Got Life Insurance?

One sunny morning, back when we were nomads hunkering down at my FIL's, Micah and I were having a conversation with him, and it went something like this:

Micah: Hey, Dad, did you or Mom ever have any life insurance policies in the past?

Dad: No! Of course not! My kids would kill me for it!

Micah: Well, it can help. Juliet's mom had a policy that helped us buy our townhouse.

Actually, this wasn't entirely accurate. My mother passed away, and I inherited the Nissan Juke because my father didn't want to drive it (although it hadn't been paid off yet, so I still had to pay off my father's loan every month). I sold my Scion TC and used the cash to decrease Micah's debt-to-income ratio, which allowed him to qualify for the townhouse. I was still in my PhD program, so I had no income. Thus, acquiring my mother's car allowed me to sell mine, which eventually assisted us in purchasing our townhouse.

Me: Ya, the prices of houses are astronomical. No one can afford anything unless they get help from their parents. Plus, many can't even pay off their student loans. It's a vicious cycle.

Stepmother-in-law chimed in: I received an inheritance from my grandmother, which helped me get my first house.

My FIL no longer had further arguments after his second wife added her two cents, which coincided with our sentiments. The practice of generational wealth was pretty much everything regarding future generations' success or at least alleviating some of their hardships.

I heard a story about a mom who was set to inherit a fortune and planned to spend all the money before she died, leaving nothing to her kids, yet she would rather donate it all to charity. Her thought was that generational wealth was not a good thing. She had experiences with friends who were hedge fund babies who had the worst work ethics and ended up being super unproductive. They lived their whole lives knowing they had a cushion. This mom didn't want her children to have this sense of financial security and be lazy. What's even more hypocritical is she herself had this financial cushion that she wanted to tear away from her own kids. It's very odd that she felt that her children did not deserve the same grace or comfort. This was a very non-empathetic way of thinking and quite greedy. It reminded me of the boomer sentiment of "pick yourself up by your bootstraps," which is entirely out of touch. Don't get me wrong, I plan on instilling financial responsibility and the value of money in my child. However, I understand the benefit of an inheritance and how it helps support future generations and beyond. Many people struggle financially, and it's a stressful situation to be in. I know a few people who grew up thinking they were dirt poor (their parents were extremely frugal and Chinese), and basically had their childhoods robbed because they were treated like adults who had to work hard. Their hustle was real and ingrained, but was this fair to them? Due to the trauma, one friend pretty much disowned their parents, and the resentment was pretty toxic and quite unhealthy. The other friend had a younger sibling who was never treated in such a manner, even received help with student debt, and had a new car to drive. The difference in treatment was drastic and quite hurtful for my friend.

Micah's family is a large one, with seven members altogether. Some were struggling and had financial issues or were dependent on their spouse. When his mother passed away back in 2011, she did not have a life insurance policy, which would have benefited the entire family. My mother reminded me at least once a month how she would leave money for me when she died. I am unsure how or why she felt the need to do this. Perhaps she saw examples from her Westernized friends and colleagues who had parents who left an inheritance. I believe my mother wanted the best for me in every way and would continue supporting my livelihood even after she was gone. This mode of thinking, combined with prioritizing education, was why I earned four degrees, secured a stable career, and developed financial common sense. My mother instilled this in me, and I cannot thank her enough.

In today's economically unstable world, generational wealth is necessary for achieving success and stability. The sentiment that the rich get richer is very true; wealth allows for peace of mind and better self-care, producing a healthy and able individual. And health equals wealth. There is more to life than working hard, and I plan on leaving my children all I can to support them, my grandkids, and my great-grandkids. The struggle is commendable yet not pretty. The strain, stress, and trauma that form both mentally and physically are passed on to future generations. Why make it more challenging than it already is? Tough love doesn't work. Punishing people for their debt doesn't prove anything.

You Come First, Always

My SIL wasn't feeling well for about five days before she finally made an appointment to see a doctor. She knew something was wrong and demanded to get a CT scan because the doctor didn't think she needed one. The scan showcased that her appendix had exploded, and her blood tests indicated multiple types of bacteria causing blood infection, aka sepsis. They put her on IV antibiotics, and she was in the hospital for over a week. She got discharged and had to clear the infection entirely before she could get surgery to remove the ruptured appendix. She asked Micah if she could stay at our place for a little while because her flat needed to be cleaned properly, and her roommate wouldn't be home to help assist her. She was not entirely disabled but would need help with certain everyday things.

I had a discussion with Micah about her staying, and initially, she said she would only stay for a few nights, but then Micah felt that she would need to stay for a couple of weeks. He thought that it was his brotherly duty to care for her since she was not well and thought we were the only ones out of his other five siblings who had the best setup for this i.e. guest bedroom and large house. I agreed that we were most likely the best option, but I didn't have much bandwidth for this household modification, even if it was temporary. I worked from home, had a toddler running around, and was working diligently to ensure my fertility was ideal and at its highest capacity. Plus, we had to schedule sperm injection nights, aka sex. Truly, I could only spend my energy on so many things that if anything threw me off my path or calendar, I would have a nervous breakdown. I didn't have the mental capacity or physical energy to add any more to my overflowing plate.

I choose myself over anyone else as I love myself the most. I am my first priority because I have a family to care for. I cannot risk my overall well-being for others because I have a career, a monthly mortgage, two dogs, a husband, a child, a social life, and a book I need to finish writing. Plus, if mummy isn't happy, no one in the house is. I told Micah a week max because I didn't want our partnership to be affected by other unnecessary stressors. He agreed.

There was a story about how a person's SIL was a functioning drug addict and asked to live with them for a while. The SIL worked in the evenings and needed a ride to and from work during the week, but her workplace was not nearby. The husband, who worked full-time, suggested that she help with pick-up and other errands during the day since she was a stay-at-home mom (SAHM) who had at least half a day free since their child went to daycare part-time. This person mentioned that she cherished her free time and was reluctant to give it up for her SIL. Her husband felt he had an older brother's duty to care for his younger sister, and they also didn't see family much because they lived far away. He even played the "if this happened to your siblings" card, and the wife stated that she would also say no to her siblings. He also believed that his sister would be distanced enough from drug dealers, which was pretty naive. Drug addicts will always find a way, plus there are dealers that will drive out long distances.

The way I see it, her home is not a drug treatment center and that both she and her husband were not equipped to take care of an addict, especially with a child to care for. What if their child accidentally got a hold of the drugs, which unfortunately occurs way too often and has a high potential for ending in death. I become sick to my stomach when I see news about toddlers dying from accidental fentanyl consumption. It's frightening how common this occurs.

I actually had an ex-boyfriend who was a drug addict, and it was the worst time of my life (except for the first six months when we were falling in love, and he wasn't yet an addict). Trying to love someone and cure them of their addiction at the same time is a fool's quest. I was riding a rollercoaster for almost four years of my life with this person because I thought I could cure him of his addiction with love. I was naive in thinking that only my love could pull someone out of their black hole. I knew jack all about how to deal with addicts and definitely did not have the tools to navigate through this tumultuous time. I don't think anyone truly can deal with a loved one's dependency on drugs. I still have nightmares about being with this person and probably developed some PTSD (post-traumatic stress disorder).

Going back to caring for a family member inside of my own home, I would not be able to do that for any of my family members, nor should they expect that of me because I am not a nurse or a caretaker. I would have to put them in a long-term care facility where they could receive the proper care they needed. Helen Hoang, an author who is known for creating characters who are on the autistic spectrum, wrote a fictitious novel called *The Heart Principle*, which incorporates autobiographical experiences. The story goes deep into Asian family dysfunction along with caring for a bedridden parent. It's raw, steamy (yes, she includes sex in type), and quite eye-opening. I learned a lot about Asperger's and the anxiety that comes along with it. It's a must-read since Helen is Asian and a mother. There is much to relate to.

The main point of this whole topic is if you do not put yourself first, your physical health and mental well-being will diminish, which cascades down to everyone who counts on you. Prolonged self-sacrifice is detrimental, unsustainable, and overrated. "Selfishness" aids in preserving sanity and is essential for acts of selflessness.

33. Give Me Back My Money

I made an appointment to consult with a new fertility specialist in Bellevue, Washington. I thought I would try Oregon Reproductive Medicine (ORM) as they were closer to me than SRM, which performs all of its major procedures in Seattle. Their Bellevue office was more limited. ORM had a policy where I was required to pay a $100 deposit for the initial consultation, which would be credited to my account. Initially, I had a bit of an issue with this, but I went along anyway. My virtual meeting was scheduled to take place at 12:30 pm, but it had already been pushed back by half an hour due to the doctor's schedule. Due to the pandemic, virtual meetings were scheduled back-to-back, and I had a work meeting that was added at the last minute, which meant I would probably be late because there was an overlap at 1 pm. So, I was waiting in Zoom for this meeting to start, and nine minutes passed with no word. I then texted the office, but there was nothing. I grew impatient and a bit furious because no one had contacted me to notify me of the doctor's whereabouts. I then called the office, and the admin person said she'd try to figure out where my doctor was and call me back. She called back and told me that my doctor was coming soon and that she was still in surgery. I began to feel quite upset and frustrated that I waited a month to talk to this doc, waited fifteen minutes for someone to tell me what the eff was going on, and now I had to worry about my next work meeting. Plus, I was about to get my period, so I was all sorts of hormonal. I told the admin person that I didn't have time to wait on people and that I had a career I had to attend to. At this point, I was almost in tears. I canceled the meeting and demanded a refund. She apologized and said she would process the refund.

I received an email from the fertility doctor apologizing and explaining the reason for the delay. If I were at the office in person, I probably wouldn't have left because someone would have notified me that the doc would be late. Perhaps I felt incredibly lonely in the Zoom waiting room, thinking no one would ever start the virtual meeting. I suppose the impersonal and empty void of virtual couldn't fully replace the dynamics of in-person meetings. A friendly assistant would have knocked on the door at the office and spoken directly to me, all with a warm smile. The cold, robotic computer screen displaying the message that someone would let me in shortly was precisely as described—cold and robotic. Fertility assistance is highly personal. If prospective mothers aren't treated with the utmost care and delicateness, things can crumble quickly. The serendipitous aspect of this experience was that I had reservations about going to a new office, and I guess they made the right decision for me. BTW, my period came two days after this appointment.

WWYD (What Would You Do?)

I reflected on a situation that occurred about seven years ago with a family member, and I wanted to write an anonymous post about it to gain some insight. Something that came to light was that these Facebook groups were not always a safe platform for venting or asking for advice. I not only witnessed this, but I also experienced it firsthand one evening. I wanted to ask the group what they would do in a certain situation involving a family member. Naively, I thought most would understand my situation, but I was disillusioned when I read comments from those who either didn't want to know where I was coming from or didn't really care to understand and just wanted to troll. Also, there was only so much one could go into detail on these posts. My post was about a family member I had blogged about in 2015 while on vacation in Vietnam. I wrote about their trauma because they had spontaneously lashed out at me after they were triggered. I will not go into great detail about the incident because it's still precarious, and the drama/trauma still lingers. What I will add is that I had no idea what I did was a trigger, nor was it directed towards them at all; in fact, it was an ordinary moment I had with a stray dog that I wanted to pet. Thus, it literally had nothing to do with how I behaved with this person; it was a completely random action that set them off. I have not communicated with this family member since the incident, and recently felt the need to clear the air. So, I apologized via email after all this time, but apparently, that was not enough. For this family member to properly move on, they requested that I apologize on my blog. My mind was going back and forth on this request. I felt it was a bit of a demand and felt no reciprocation on their end in actually mending the broken relationship. It was as if I were the only person at fault in this charade, and the other person felt no need to be accountable for their actions.

I asked the online group what they thought I should do. From the poll, there were 1,124 votes and 164 comments. Just over 50% said I should apologize on my blog. Some comments were supportive, and there were unsupportive ones, too, that cut pretty deep, even if they weren't accurate. Readers, unfortunately, do not receive all the context and nuances within the dynamic; thus, they can only react subjectively after reading your post based on their emotions. I am a blunt and sarcastic individual, and this didn't sit well with some people. I suppose delivery was everything, but people want sugarcoating, and that's just not me. I came out of this experience a little shaken, and then reflected on how famous people felt when smear campaigns or rumors were published about them. My empathy for those in the spotlight has increased, and now I can see why Kelly Marie Tran, who starred in Star Wars: Episode VIII, The Last Jedi, left social media due to the horrible posts and reactions to her being in the film. Even Constance Wu, who couldn't even speak her truth without having her words misconstrued, had to take a break for a few years. Even when you aren't putting yourself out there, the internet has ways of displaying you in a format you did not intend. That was the lesson I learned from blogging about my family member in 2015 when I believed I was venting my truth, which I was, but not without consequence. I was wrong to write about someone else's triggers, and after my experience posting in this group, I wrote a simple apology on my blog (by the way, I had always intended to do this, even before I posted about it on the group page). I still have not heard back from this family member, but things take time, and maybe we can all move past this once and for all. And even if this person still cannot move forward, I have done all I can, and I feel redeemed by that.

I Told You to Go See a Doctor!

It was exactly 8 pm on November 14, 2022. I was awaiting word from Micah, who had just checked himself into the emergency hospital in Issaquah. A few weeks ago, he complained about feeling lightheaded and dizzy. Then, he caught the cold I gave Tobin, so we thought it was the virus, possibly RSV. This past weekend, he felt off, and I told him to either see the doctor or use Teledoc. He had way worse symptoms compared to Tobin and me, and may have developed an upper respiratory tract infection as his sinuses were causing quite a bit of pain. He finally connected with Teledoc, and they prescribed him antibiotics. He recently received a botched haircut, so he went to Issaquah for a buzz cut because he hated it so much and wanted to start over. I received a call around 3:30 pm, and Micah reported that the hair stylist had just called an ambulance because he was beginning to feel tingly in his arms and at the back of his head. He was pretty out of it. I asked him where they would take him, and he didn't know, maybe Swedish Hospital. He had to hang up because the EMT was there to assess him. About twenty-five minutes later, he called me back, and the EMT told him to go to urgent care to get screened and have his blood work done. They also mentioned that he probably should not have been driving. I had to pick up Tobin from daycare, so we met at Dough Zone, located in the same parking lot as the barbershop. Micah hadn't had lunch yet and was hungry. He continued to rest for a bit and then drove our Subaru through the parking lot to the restaurant.

Micah was ravenous and over-ordered, of course. I put Tobin in his high chair, and within five minutes, the waitress served us two bowls of dan dan noodles, two steamed baskets of pork xiao long bao, a plate of q-baos, chicken dumplings in soup, and the sweet & sour squiggly cucumber.

"I may have overdone it," Micah said. Over dinner, he said he had never felt these tingly sensations before and was very anxious. His hairstylist wasn't helping either to soothe his fears. I asked him if he thought this was it when he was waiting for the ambulance, and he said yes. I told him I couldn't care for the toddler without him. He laughed because he thought I said I couldn't care of the garden without him.

"Ya, that too," I said. This past month, he created a masterpiece with our landscape and pathways, driving back and forth to two different rock suppliers to purchase a variety of gravel and the salt and pepper quartz bricks I had picked out to line the paths. It had been pretty strenuous on his body, all of the physical labor, but he was on a mission to finish before the ground froze. This morning, we saw frost.

After dinner, Micah went to urgent care, and I took Tobin home to prepare for bedtime. I received a call around 7 pm, and Micah mentioned that the doctor at the urgent care facility had performed an EKG. He was concerned with the results and advised him to go to the emergency room, as the diagnosis was beyond his pay grade. I was like, excuse me? So essentially, he ended up in an emergency anyway! The bloody EMT person should have just taken him there in the first place! Thus, Micah drove up the hill to check himself in and said he would update me.

I didn't know what to do with myself, so I put the Pottery Barn duvet cover back on our king-size duvet. The fabric is a woven, checked black and white pattern, which snagged easily if you had a Shiba Inu named Tomtom scratching at it every other night to make her bed. I used the post of my earring to poke the pulled-out threads back into the linen weave. I had moments of worry and shock ebbing in and out of my head like ocean waves. The shock can be debilitating and put you in a trance for a moment, and then you can continue to complete the task at hand. Micah texted me to let me know that the emergency room was full and he wouldn't be home anytime soon. He told me he wanted to be at home in bed, snuggling with me, and that he was worried. I told him not to stress too much and that I loved him. I texted some friends to let them know, and they offered to help me if I needed anything.

Relief

I was getting ready for bed when I received a text from Micah saying he was driving home. It was just past 11 pm. I was thankful he was coming home and anxious to hear how the rest of his time went at the emergency room. Once he got home, he told me that the doctor had run another EKG, blood tests, and a COVID test. All came out negative, and there didn't seem to be any issues. They suggested he follow up with his primary care physician. Micah was so confused as to why he experienced all the symptoms he did, and there seemed to be nothing wrong. The nurse said perhaps it was an anxiety attack or the virus that he caught was causing the dizzy spells. We were glad he didn't have to stay the night there. I was so relieved he was okay for now and safe at home. We had a bit of a scare, and hopefully, that would be the last of it. However, we still needed to figure out what the health issues were. I wondered if long COVID would present itself after being gone for so long.

<u>Friends Forever?</u>

So I have this one friend, Elaine, whom I knew pretty early on when I moved to Seattle. Thus, we have a relatively long history and have tried to be there for one another at birthday parties and life-changing events, such as weddings and baby showers. We didn't hang out regularly, even though we were flat neighbors at one point for a few years. She literally lived down the hall from me. I believe one of the reasons why Elaine wanted to continue our friendship was because she wanted her boyfriend to connect with Micah so they could be like best buddies or something since they are both white and maybe could relate. Who knows. Everyone loves Micah and thinks he is a great guy, and he gets along with everyone, even if he disagrees with their values. I believe that is one thing I love about him, and he made it easy for my friends to accept him and support our relationship. As time passed, Elaine had a few kids, and I saw less of her. At best, we saw each other a couple times a year, but we went to their wedding, which was out of town.

In the summer of 2020, during the first year of the pandemic, right at the tail end of the first peak, Black Lives Matter (BLM) protests broke out, and Seattle's Capitol Hill on 12th and Pine was the epicenter of chaos and violence. Tear gas, flashbangs, and pepper spray were the methods used by Seattle Police to quell non-violent protests. It was mayhem. One day, Elaine and I got into it during the height of BLM, when tension and divisive politics ran high. Over the years, it seemed Elaine was becoming more conservative in mindset, and it showcased when we exchanged texts on vaccines - her stance was pretty much anti-vaxxer. She even shared with me YouTube videos of COVID conspiracies and how the hospitals were labeling non-COVID deaths as COVID-related (by the way, COVID can cause secondary illness or exacerbate chronic conditions, which leads to other types of fatalities but are still considered COVID-related). She seemed to be drinking the Fox News Kool-Aid that her husband was feeding her, and I was like, "Who are you?" So we had a blown-out text argument because I was waving my big bloody BLM flag, and she was waving her All Lives Matter flag. She even told me that she gave gifts to Black families in need every Christmas, which had no direct correlation to being woke. Elaine couldn't understand why I was for defunding the police and why I wanted money to be used for more helpful services like mental health case workers. It was a messy debate with her putting words in my mouth, and I was surprised she even showed up at my baby shower three months after this. Mind you, she was late as usual, which was annoying.

After we had settled into our new house, I tried to make plans to hang out a few times with Elaine. I was very concerned because she had stopped posting entirely on social media. Thus, I reached out numerous times this past Spring, Summer, and Fall to reconnect, but my efforts were not met with the same type of reciprocation, or at least if they were, it wasn't entirely genuine on her end because we failed to meet. I grew weary of constantly reaching out; thinking about our dissolved friendship was mentally draining. Then, one day, I was on a tea date with a couple of my gfs and brought up Elaine. My gf, who also has a white husband and kids around the same age as Elaine, was invited over for a fabulous dinner about a month ago. I was like, "Excuse me?" My gf noticed I was visibly aghast that she hung out with Elaine, where my efforts were rejected, she tried to soften the situation by adding that their kids were similar in age, so she probably wanted them to bond. Again, here was another example of how Elaine would rather be friends with someone she could benefit from or whom her loved ones could connect with. I am not saying this is a bad thing; it's just something I noticed, and I don't value it. I care for my gfs a great deal. Thus, for all of my close longtime friends, I am very intentional in sustaining the relationship regardless of how our lives change over the years. I am friends with them, NOT their partners or children. This brings me to another irritating factor I have with close friends who have kids - they will connect and contact you more often if your kids are closer in age. I get it, but now I don't get to hang out with my longtime friend. Instead, she plans to hang out with my other close girlfriend and invites her over to hang out! The other thing to note is that I introduced Elaine to my gf a few years back because they were at my events. So Elaine basically stole my friend, who was apparently more hang-out-worthy since they both have white husbands and kids who are around the same age and was rejecting my friendship because I stood for BLM and wanted police reform.

That night I changed the Netflix password and deleted their profile. #salty

34. My Father

I had been feeling some daughter guilt as of late because I preferred not to visit my father for Christmas. I just didn't have the energy to do the drive up, pack the toddler and the dogs, rent an Airbnb, and wait in line at the border for who knows how long (by the way, Tobin didn't have a Nexus, so the wait would have been even longer), all to have lunch with my dad. But then, when my friends told me my dad was old, and I should try to spend as much time with him as possible, or when they mentioned planning fun trips with their mothers, I felt even more guilty. Then I'd remember how fussy my toddler would be in his car seat for six bloody hours (roundtrip), and I would feel better about the situation. Since Tobin was so mobile, it would be torture for him to be strapped down for so long, and he probably had the same sentiment, which was evident by the noisy 15-minute ride back home from daycare. My bandwidth for any extraneous activity is almost non-existent. Thinking about anything other than work and home life has made me want to nap. Thus, it was settled, and I wasn't seeing my father and half-sister during the winter holiday. My dad doesn't like traveling anymore because he is old. I hope he liked the West Coast-themed gift basket that was delivered just before his birthday. I know it wasn't the same, but I was so beat.

My father is an interesting character, to say the least. I grew up watching him type independent journalistic articles, cut up pieces to produce a magazine layout and adhere to a makeshift booklet with a glue stick. His Viet newspaper was simple and primitive, yet the voice that resonated from the pages was fierce. Phuoc Dang is a patriotic and proud man, posting his large yellow flag with the three red stripes on top of our house. I was utterly embarrassed by it, perhaps because I wanted assimilation and to be like all the other white people in our community, which comprised of many Jewish people. Coincidentally, I ended up dating two Jewish men and unfortunately broke their latke-loving hearts.

I love Jewish men; they possess my two favorite traits - intellect and humor.

Many are well-traveled, cultured, and value family. What more could you ask for, right? Well, let me tell you, the thing you need to fear are the women in their lives who could rip you apart and love you to death at the same time. Even though I had some hostile moments with some of these women, I miss how I was treated like family after we got through some of the growing pains. Both of my exes had a hard time bringing me in because I wasn't Jewish or white. However, after all the fuss, their families came to love me, and I loved them. Their family dynamics were so different from my own. There were never any secrets; everything was out in the open. I do remember quite a bit of yelling and fighting. Yet the family was tight-knit, and the emotional availability was infinite. I greatly cherished this since I grew up alone as an only child.

So, back to my father, the voice of reason for Vietnam, who believed Americans came to help them win the war. When I was growing up, I was told I had a half-sister. One summer, while visiting cousins in Windsor, Ontario, my closest cousin divulged that I had more half-siblings—a brother and another sister. I was shocked, but it didn't end there. As I became closer to my half-sister, who resides in Vancouver, it became apparent through stories that my father was not a monogamous partner. He left a set of male twins behind, and who knew how many other biological children there were? It was both impressive and repulsive all at once.

My father was spreading his seeds as he pleased with no repercussions. Maybe I was envious because I would love to share my DNA with the world and create a dynasty, just like Elon Musk and his father (I kid). My father's relationship with many of his children was essentially estranged. He spoke to my half-sister and half-brother, but another half-sister did not talk to him. I believe it was a tough time when he left his first family. I got quite a bit of controversial stories from other family members, and it affected how I felt about him, although it is transient because he's still my father. I only know my experiences with him. There were stories of him taking money from his sisters before he fled Vietnam. I do not know if that happened or if he borrowed the cash to escape the country. Perhaps I should give him the benefit of the doubt. It's so easy for people to say, "Well, why don't you ask him?" That's complicated, too.

My relationship with my father revolved around essentially two sentences:

"How are you?"

"How's the weather?"

I don't speak Vietnamese, and his English is very limited. Thus, we don't go deep at all when conversing. I need to learn Viet soon, but where do I find the time and energy? Even if I did learn, the dynamics between my father and I are very surface-level anyhow. After my mother passed in 2014, and as he ages, it became more challenging to communicate with him when he needed assistance. Either he didn't fully understand what I said, or if he did, he did his own thing anyway. Old people can be difficult to deal with, especially refugees with PTSD from the war. I tried my best to connect with him, and he was happy when we'd video chat with Tobin. I am the last child he had, but who knows what sort of information will surface with time? Even with his flaws, my father was a constant in my life, and I had stability and love. Thus, that is something for which I am very grateful. Children tend to imitate what they see at home, and watching my father type away for his newspaper was exactly what I was doing then. My mother always said, "Like father, like daughter."

35. My Mother

When I became a mother, reflecting on my experiences with my mother was natural. There came an understanding of why my mom was so strict and why she loved me deeply, even though it was pretty irritating. As an only child, it was hard not to feel suffocated by my parents' constant hovering. I was loved unconditionally, which was rare in Vietnamese households, so I've heard. My mother allowed me to take on any desired extracurricular activities - ballet, piano, flute. My highest priority was my education; I am grateful for this discipline.

Nga Thai was from Da Lat, a mountainous region of Vietnam where coffee beans and tea bushes grow. She told me that nuns taught her how to speak and read English, which was interesting, though she did not follow the faith and continued to adhere to Buddhist practices. I don't know very much about her past because these details were never divulged to me, and my mom passed away suddenly in 2014 due to a brain aneurysm. From our family vault of secrets, I was told she was my father's mistress before they both fled Vietnam in a boat and landed on the shores of a beach in Thailand. My philandering father must have seen an opportunity with my mother since she spoke English and was willing to flee the country with him. Maybe he thought escaping with his original three children and wife would be extremely risky along with being too dangerous. Or, perhaps, he was just thinking of himself. Who knows. Either way, their destiny was to escape together and have me. They lived on the beaches of Thailand for a few months before being sponsored to Winnipeg, MB, Canada, in 1980. I came a year later.

My mother was a homebody and couldn't understand why I always wanted to be out and about. She was content with her work schedule, cooking, cleaning, and watching TV. Or, at least, it seemed like she was content with her life. I honestly did not have a clue. All I knew was that she didn't go anywhere out of the country, and she wanted the best life for me. Thus, she did everything in her power to give me a stable home life. I don't have any regrets, but I carry some for my mother. She would always say, "Work now, play later." She held some fantasy that she could travel the world once she retired. But who would have the energy at age 65 to travel like someone 40 years younger? She was a work horse her whole life, a dedicated first-grade teacher who never set foot on a plane to Europe. I remember her reading French books and reciting them aloud. If only she had the foresight to know she would die after she retired and never have the chance to travel internationally. I wonder how things would have turned out. I found this a morbidly fatal irony, and my heart broke for her. It became my duty to show her the world through my eyes and physically sprinkle her ashes in Greece, Switzerland, Vietnam, Norway, Malta, Kauai, and other international locations. My mum got to travel the world, but only as dust.

My mother and I had a tumultuous relationship while I was growing up. Being an only child was difficult because all eyes were on me all the bloody time. Even though she loved me unconditionally, it was all too much with the nagging and helicopering. We fought often, and it probably wasn't about anything important. I didn't have siblings to fight with, so I did it with my mom. It's like I thought I was on my own debate team and needed to prove my mother wrong every time, no matter the topic. It was exhausting and dysfunctional. We were never close like she wished us to be, and I felt terrible about that. However, she created a certain dynamic between us that was very much parent dictates child, where she was always right, where I had to listen to her even if I could prove her wrong. Perhaps this was why I was so disrespectful. I was rebelling against her authority, which I found to be suffocating. The word "no" became a trigger for me, and I carried it outside of the house. Even at institutions outside my home, such as university, I lashed out against authoritative figures. For example, if I were absent or late to class and had professors ask me where I was or what I was doing, I would give attitude and say something rude like, "None of your business."

My behavior transferred to other places and relationships. It was an outward projection, essentially my way of being free of the strict matriarchal shackles thrust upon me. Even still, my mother was a constant in my life, and I was fearless in the world because she was my rock and safety net no matter what. I never had to doubt her love and care for me ever. However, these feelings of invincibility, if you will, dissipated during her sudden death. My constant was no longer there, and I began to fear the unknown. My grief transformed into bouts of depression where I didn't feel joy in certain things, such as international travel plans or moving into our new townhouse. The thought of not being able to share these milestones with my mother numbed me.

There were a variety of items I had to deal with besides grieving over my mother. All of the funeral and cremation details I had to decide on were not good enough for my aunt and uncle, who were mad at me because they weren't able to watch her body get cremated. The body was sent to another building across the US border, which I had no clue of, nor did I ever think anyone would want to watch her body being thrown into the incinerator. I had to deal with transferring my parents' car into my name because my father didn't want to drive in Vancouver. And then there was all the banking. Money is venom for all relationships; people can be weird and petty about such matters. At first, I had access to all my father's accounts to ensure his bills were all paid and everything was in order. Then, one day, I couldn't access his online account. I was on the phone with him, trying to let him know I was only there to help him, and we argued. The language barrier was already a huge struggle, so it was tough to communicate anything with him properly. Then, I received a call from my cousin saying that my father had been telling his side of the family that I had been taking money from him, which was ludicrous. The fact was, I didn't need nor did I ever need any of his money. The other part was that it wasn't even his money but my mother's money. I felt I had a fiduciary responsibility towards my father because he was old and not thinking straight at all after the death of my mother. Plus, my mom dealt with all the finances, so he knew nothing or very little. My mom was pretty much the nucleus when it came to the family relationships, and now apoptosis had occurred, damaging all family lines. I had barely enough energy to defend myself, yet it did not matter if I had the best defense speech of my life. People believed what they wanted to believe. Every single one of my actions during the year of her death was criticized. It was blasphemous that I purchased my first townhouse (not that it was anyone's business, but Micah and I did this on our own without external help), that I went on vacation to Europe in the Fall, and then planned a wedding for the end of the year. My family did not want me to live my life to the fullest because I was supposed to be grieving for a whole bloody year. Was this some Vietnamese practice

I was never told about? I had no clue. I was utterly ignorant of what to do when my mom died and everyone blamed me for it. I had been estranged. I was the lone wolf, even more so. Dealing with all of the tedious tasks of a loved one's death while grieving was pretty much a curse that I never want to experience again, but I know that one day again it will be inevitable.

Secrets from the grave are a real thing. I had no clue I would ever experience this, but while going through my mother's documents, I found a photo of her with a young child, probably around the age of three. Along with the picture were two birth certificates—one for a child and one for the child's father. Essentially, I found out that my mom had a daughter who was six years older than me. This took me back to a memory I had of my mom. We were watching Sally Field's film *Not Without My Daughter*, and my mom mentioned how she would never leave her child behind. I was probably nine then and little did I know she was speaking from experience. I learned about the situation from my cousin, who questioned her mother (my mom's sister). The father of this child found out that my mother was having an affair with my dad and took their daughter away. Looking back, I realized that when I thought my mother was speaking about my half-sister on my dad's side, she may have been indirectly speaking about her own daughter. It brought tears to my eyes, knowing I could never inquire about this with my mom, and it is entirely unfortunate that she never told me. The only clue she gave me was that she had a secret she would tell me on her deathbed. My mom was so weird. As a teenager at the time, I was like, "Whatever, Mom." I find the secrets that have been kept from me incredible. And to what? Protect me? From what, exactly? The truth? I have completed three different DNA tests to maybe one day have a match with my lost half-sibling. Does she even know she has other family? What did her father say about our mother? Is she safe? Is she even alive? So many unanswered questions.

What made me the saddest about my mother's death was thinking how she would never get to know her grandson. Same with my mother-in-law, who died in 2011. Our mothers are goddesses; we will continue to worship them and make sure Tobin knows all about his incredible grandmothers.

36. Round Two of IVF?

We tried getting pregnant when Tobin was around the one-year mark. When he turned two, I was still not pregnant. Like the first round, I prepped my body, although not as rigorously - I saw my acupuncturist every other week, took my supplements, and tried to eat "warming" foods. We had a virtual consult with the same fertility doc as last time, and she was so happy to hear that Tobin was healthy, growing, and just the sweetest toddler. I told her I was grateful to have such an excellent, supportive, and professional doctor. It made her day to hear that.

Dr. Bird laid out all of the realistic scenarios we could encounter and the limited options I would have due to my age. I was turning forty-two. Thus, the success rate was less than when I was about to turn thirty-nine. We discussed that a fresh embryo transfer would be best again, but perhaps waiting for the embryos to develop until day five (the last time I transferred at day three), because if something were wrong, the embryo would not survive genetically. We were leaving it up to nature instead of poking the embryos to test them. I was scheduled to do a hysteroscopy, an ultrasound of my ovaries, and some blood tests. According to Dr. Bird, the hysteroscopy should be a cake walk since I had a vaginal birth. The timing of my cycle had to be between days 5-12, and I had work travel to Boise during that same week. A cancellation popped up, but I was flying out that same day, so they told me to call back the day I would be flying back home. Fortunately, I got an appointment on day 12 of my cycle at the last minute.

On the day of my appointment, I exited on Mercer off of I-5 and headed towards Westlake. Seeing Lake Union and the area brought back memories of my visits to SRM. I again felt a sense of importance being back working on another "project." The office was still not allowing partners to join the appointments, which was disappointing because I would have thought things would be back to normal. I suppose they wanted to continue COVID mitigation and strict policy to protect the prospective mothers. I was back in the familiar ultrasound room, where I undressed from the waist down, sat on a reclining chair, covered myself with the sheet, and waited. Since I was on day 12, I was excited to see if any follicles were developing. Three people entered the room after a knock on the door. It seemed like one was a more experienced tech, one was the newer tech, and the other an assistant. The newer tech was a WOC, and I always appreciated diversity. She explained everything she was going to do. The first part was the ultrasound, and I had a dominant follicle developing in my left ovary. It looked like about three other follicles were present as well. This was a good sign, and I was happy that my ovaries were still working. The next part was the hysteroscopy, where they stuck a little camera up my cervix to view my uterine cavity and fallopian tubes. It was a little crampy, and they had to shoot water up my cervix for the camera to have a proper view. It was very cool to look at the inside of my reproductive tract. They even zoomed into the openings of my fallopian tubes, which looked clear and healthy. The tech counted down from three, and when one came around, she pulled out the scope, and all of this water came gushing out of my vagina. It probably made a huge mess because the more experienced tech came over and began putting more absorbent pads on the ground and one under my butt. Overall, my reproductive organs looked healthy. Yay!

Micah made an appointment to have his sperm analyzed, and they were booking after the new year already, which was a month away. I groaned because I wanted to know if everything was okay on his end, and he began to respond in the "I told you I should have made an appointment sooner" manner. I told him he was right for once, but how did I know there would be a backlog in the sperm department?

<u>Monkey See, Monkey Do</u>

I was on my flight back from Sacramento, my last work trip of the year, and during our ascent into the cool evening air, I noticed the woman in the aisle seat to my right and one row up pushing the button for the flight attendant. She asked for a bag and then spit in a cup she was holding. I was like, oh my god, she is about to ralph. I averted my eyes but, from my peripheral vision, witnessed the flight attendant running as fast as she could with a garbage bag. She didn't make it on time, so barf had splattered in the aisle. I didn't see it because my eyes closed, but the attendant returned with some coffee grinds, sprinkled them on the carpet, and laid some absorbent pads down. I have a pretty queasy stomach, and I just prayed that I wouldn't get airsick with all the commotion. I also felt terrible for the lady but then stopped feeling bad after another flight attendant came by to assess the situation. She asked the ill lady if she had been drinking alcohol, and the lady nodded her head. Thus, much of this probably could have been prevented. The flight attendant told her she needed to hydrate and eat some snacks. About twenty minutes later, the garbage bag was filling up again, making me shut my eyes immediately.

I was thankful I had my mask on and couldn't smell anything foul. The attendant took the soupy bag and replaced it with another one. I thought I was going to lose it. I tried to distract myself with the book I had just purchased, *Daughters of the New Year*, by E.M. Tran. My Viet author collection had multiplied this year, and I just finished *House of Sticks* by Ly Ky Tran; it was so raw and honest. This new wave of women Viet authors was impressive and so inspirational. And, yet, I digress. I landed back in Seattle without tossing my cookies. Thank god. However, this was only the beginning of a very disagreeable weekend ahead.

The following day, we were getting Tobin ready for daycare, but he threw up and had diarrhea, so he had to stay home. We were hoping he ate something bad, but after we fed him a bit more food, it all came back up again, and I knew it was viral gastroenteritis (most people call it stomach flu even though it has nothing to do with the flu virus). After calling Teladoc, I found that there was a regimen of no solids and mainly fluids for the next day or so. We were also told orange juice was very acidic, so we did not give him that. After a few days, he seemed to be better, but then, Saturday night, he barfed right after we put him to bed. After cleaning him up and getting ready for bed again, we put him down again. About five minutes later, we heard him wailing and saying, "Oh no!" repeatedly. Poor guy, he was so traumatized with all of the vomiting. We tried to console him and tell him everything was okay and that mommy and daddy would clean it up. We finally cleaned him up, put him down the third time, and prayed he wouldn't have another episode. I then began to feel ill to my stomach and wondered if I had caught his virus or if it was just uneasiness from all the chaos and cleaning up. I went to lie down in bed, and then I began to feel quite nauseous. I dragged myself to the bathroom with some plastic bags, but it was not a pretty sight. I still had my Thai food in a bowl to finish. That was not going to happen. I realized that witnessing the lady on the plane foreshadowed what was to come. Micah slept in the guest room to give me privacy if I needed to ralph more. I probably threw up four to five times within five hours. I was so exhausted with the retching. A plastic bag was placed right under my cheek as I lay paralyzed due to nausea. It reminded me of my delivery, where I would toss my cookies after every cycle of contraction and pushing. It was after 1 am and I knew I needed to boost my immune system somehow. I dragged myself to the guest room and woke Micah, who was fast asleep. What I needed was Viet green ointment witchery on my back. He sprinkled the potent menthol green ointment all over my back and, using an Asian soup spoon, began to scrape my back outwardly. Not bad for only having done it a few times beforehand. My skin was even more sensitive to the illness, but I knew I needed to stimulate my immune system. I also doused my tummy with the ointment to cover all bases. It must have worked, or maybe I had some memory antibodies from a previous stomach virus and could halt further virus replication, but I did not barf anymore that night or after that. I had Micah do a few more rounds of Viet green ointment on my back during the day. My stomach was in quite a bit of pain due to the acid coming up my esophagus. I took little slips of coconut water to hydrate myself. I even took Monday off to rest another day. Tobin seemed well enough to attend daycare, so we sent him off.

When we picked him up after 4 pm, Micah wanted sushi, so we went to Kura in Bellevue. Tobin had a bit of a poop blowout at daycare but seemed to be okay, and we had to feed him before bedtime. We ordered his favorites - eel nigiri, shrimp tempura, and some fries. He seemed to be eating okay, and I looked at him and saw that he was slowing down a bit. He didn't look like he was feeling so well, and as that thought lingered in the air, it all came. He cried and repeatedly said, "Oh no!" We rushed to clean him up quickly to get him out of the restaurant.

I asked the server for a plastic bag and a wet cloth, and she told me to grab my food on the conveyor belt because the kitchen was yelling about it. It was sheer chaos. I tried to clean up the table as best as I could and tried to cover what was on the floor. I felt so bad about the other customers seeing the mess. I offered to clean the floor, too, but the server said they had protocols for that, and the highchair was an utter mess. Micah apologized for even thinking it was a good idea for us to take him out. I suppose the lesson was that even if you thought your toddler was done with his stomach virus, there may be a little more illness left. Oh, and always have a second set of clothes in your car. We practiced this when Tobin was a baby and stopped doing it as he grew. Viral gastroenteritis is the worst for all parties involved. We had to wait a bit to show our faces at our favorite sushi spot.

37. Ho Ho No!

Christmas came way too quickly. Everything was cancelled because a tripledemic occurred with flu, COVID, and RSV floating around. After my GI (gastrointestinal) virus, I not only lost a few pounds because I couldn't eat or keep anything down, but I also developed a persistent dry cough. I suppose one thing I was able to celebrate was getting into my Ted Baker size zero dress, which I never thought I would ever fit again. It was snug, but I could still zip it up! Feeling thin again felt good, and it took me two years to almost return to my original size.

Everything that could happen over the holidays did happen. In addition to all the illnesses, we had a snowstorm, an ice storm, a power outage that lasted 24 hours, and death (an acquaintance I had known since 2012 committed suicide), all while Tobin was home from daycare. Plus, we had to babysit our besties' two dogs (they were on a Zambian safari). Walking four dogs three times a day in snow and ice was not fun. Our black and tan shiba, Tomtom, who was already particular and peculiar in excreting her bodily waste, would not pee on the ice, so she decided she wouldn't pee for a bloody day. Our anxiety was through the roof, and we almost killed ourselves slipping on the ice. We had to wear micro spikes on our boots. Thank god Micah had a pair.

The suicide affected me a great deal. I am still processing it and can't pinpoint what I am feeling, but perhaps I just feel sad for this person and their family. It was a tragic and horrific death.

After speaking with others about their winter holidays, we weren't the only ones who had a bizarre week. Even with the not-very-relaxing time off, we were thankful for each other and the life we built for ourselves.

<u>Morphology</u>

It was the second day of the new year, and Micah headed to SRM in the morning for his sperm analysis. We received the results within a few days, and Micah was perplexed by one aspect of the analysis. Volume, total motile count, motility percent, and concentration seemed to be more than adequate, but the morphology was what he was concerned with. WHO gives a value of >4% for normal morphology, and Micah's result was 2%. I asked my acupuncturist to explain this data point to me. She said that 2% of his sperm were consistent with each other, but that may not mean they were necessarily "normal" looking. For example, if most looked circular, 2% were consistent with this circular shape. My fertility doctor or nurse hadn't commented on his results thus we still need to receive an explanation from them. Upon further analysis, it looked like progressive motility may be an issue as well. If this was the case, to me, that meant the sperm was not getting to my golden egg, which was so sad.

The Loma Linda Center for Fertility & IVF used the Kruger Strict Criteria to describe and evaluate sperm morphology. Here were their standards:

>14% of sperm with normal morphology = fertility is high
4-14% = fertility slightly decreased
0-3% = fertility greatly impaired

The most common cause of male infertility was low sperm count. However, the shape of the sperm played a role as well. To penetrate the egg, sperm are required to be a particular shape. Ways to overcome these issues are IUI and IVF. Within IVF, the ICSI (intracytoplasmic sperm injection) technique was quite advantageous. This was where the best-looking sperm was captured with a micro needle and inserted directly into the egg. The two embryos that I had fertilized were completed in this manner. This method was essential for those with a 0-3% morphology rating.

<u>Global Sperm Count Decline</u>

Temporal trends in sperm count: a systematic review and meta-regression analysis of samples collected globally in the 20th and 21st centuries by Levine et al. was published on November 15th, 2022, in the human reproduction update. The results demonstrated that sperm count was declining at an accelerated pace worldwide. In 1973, the estimated sperm count was 101 mill/ml; in 2018, values dropped to 49 mill/ml, which was close to a 50% decrease. The data was astonishing and should be a call for action to investigate further male fertility issues and the etiologies associated. I hypothesized that there were a variety of environmental and lifestyle habits that contributed to sperm production and quality. Factors to consider were microplastics, pesticides, alcohol and caffeine consumption, medication, unhealthy weight, stress, lack of sleep, and genetics.

According to the Loma Linda fertility website, sperm production dropped after age 40, and the sperm, unfortunately, were less robust. Here is the regimen they proposed for healthy sperm production:

- regular exercise
- avoiding steroids, tobacco, alcohol, and drugs
- reducing caffeine consumption
- healthy weight
- avoiding hot tubs
- decreasing stress
- wearing loose underwear
- consuming food/supplements rich in antioxidants

It takes approximately three months to revamp your sperm. Thus, this is a work in progress and does not occur overnight. The site suggested freezing sperm when men are young. What a bloody revelation! We have been taught that women should be the ones to preserve their eggs before their ovaries become geriatric. It seems both parties should participate in this act of reproductive cryopreservation.

Women have been the punching bags when it came to fertility issues, which I am so over. At the beginning of my IVF journey, one of my friends said to me that it was usually the woman who had the issue. I completely disagreed with this sentiment, especially after reading the latest research. If sperm count has declined by almost 50% in the last 45 years and sperm morphology is compromised, it doesn't matter what women are doing to prep their bodies because, indeed, the onus should

173

be on the man. Why was no one giving men instructions on how to prep their bodies for IVF? Is this yet another facet of patriarchal society women have to navigate through? I think my head is about to explode.

38. So Over It, Yet Not

I paid $4,689.31 upfront to SRM to move forward with an IVF cycle. My insurance would cover the rest or most of it, depending on how much the medications cost. Working on having a second child was taxing. Not only was I putting much of my time and energy into getting my body ready, but I was spending a bunch of cash to do so.

Meanwhile, my husband played video games and, by default, had more liberty to do what he pleased. Perhaps this created some bitterness not just for me, but I was bitter for all women who did all of the work while their partners didn't need to do much. I mean, our partners could try to lead healthier lives, go to acupuncture, drink less beer and coffee, or do something, anything! Maybe I was irritated because whenever I felt a mittelschmerz (ovulation cramp), I thought about the golden egg that may go to waste, for there was potential it would not get fertilized.

Micah could have done various things to help rectify his abnormal sperm morphology, which would have increased our chances of a healthy embryo forming. He wanted a second child, but how much work would he do to have one? This modified my feelings on the second journey after discovering that it may not be my issue. Essentially, I didn't feel that to have a successful, health pregnancy, IVF was the best option. All the work should not be placed on me. My exhaustion lay for all the women out there who felt the onus was on them to have a child. Men need to step up and do something. Women endure way too much, and it isn't fair. I am so done with women, myself included, believing that our bodies are the fertility issue and that, in our mid-30s, we need to adjust our habits and lifestyle. I dedicated so much of my time, energy, and money during my IVF journey, and upon reflection, I probably only needed to do 50% of the activities if someone had mentioned to me and Micah that males needed to make appropriate modifications as well. The thought of carrying a baby for nine months made me want to crawl into bed and sleep for 9 months. Was I having second thoughts? I suppose having a two-year-old toddler with his own mind didn't help the situation either. And, Tobin was one of the "good" kids as his personality was pretty happy-go-lucky.

It's Not Over Until It's Over

So, remember how I was mad at my girlfriend Elaine and changed my Netflix password? After the new year, she texted me and made plans for us to come over. She finally divulged that there was family health stuff occurring, which made it hard for her to connect with friends and get back to a more "normal" social state. So now I was the a-hole, LMFAO! I tried hard to make plans with her yet didn't feel the reciprocation nor did she ever give me a good reason as to her absence. Perhaps she didn't feel like explaining or was too exhausted; I had to understand and accept that. The lesson was that you never knew what was happening with people unless they told you. You can only do so much with the information handed to you; in this case, it wasn't given to me. We had a good time hanging out and catching up. I just wished that she had confided in me a tiny bit so I could have been there to support her. If a true friend reaches out to you, please respond and let them know what's up. You all know the repercussions if you don't - no more Netflix for you!

Asians in Film

Yesterday night was the Oscars, and to watch it, Micah signed up for the free trial for YouTube TV, so it was worth it. He canceled the subscription immediately after I watched it because the regular TV charge would be $65/month, which was a rip-off with all of the commercials. *Everything Everywhere All At Once* made history. The movie won seven out of eleven nominations, including Best Actress for Michelle Yeoh, Best Supporting Actor for Ke Huy Quan, and Best Picture. It was an incredibly monumental evening for Asians in film, where we so often play the sidekick with the "Oriental" accent. I was quite involved in the Seattle acting world, and at one point, I was the leading Asian woman chosen for multiple commercials for major companies such as Microsoft, Amazon, T-Mobile, Dell, AMD, Lenscrafters, etc. I was also in Awolnation's music video, Hollow Moon. Commercial work was more lucrative and available than film in the

Pacific Northwest. My experience was limited. So back in 2016, I decided to create my own short film, which I wrote, directed, produced, cast, and acted in. It was titled "Such Shiba. Such Wow," and it was hilariously amateur. My point in creating this short was to have an entire BIPOC cast because I was tired of the lack of diversity in Hollywood and the erasure of lead Asian roles. Then came *Crazy Rich Asians* (2018) and *Shang-Chi* (2021), which was this ginormous flag signaling to Hollywood that all-Asian casts could become blockbusters. And, of course, let's not forget *Crouching Tiger Hidden Dragon* (2000), a 23-year-old film and obsession of mine. But even before that, a film that affected me during childhood was *Joy Luck Club* (1993). This was the OG film that demonstrated the detriment and dysfunction of Asian families and was done so eloquently - the essence of Amy Tan.

Representation is essential for BIPOC communities, and now our children can watch Asian superheroes on the big screen. Experiencing the acceptance speeches from Michelle Yeoh and Ke Huy Quan was monumental and demonstrated that these actors were not past their prime.

Round Two Begins

My period began three days ago, which meant that I was on day three of my new IVF journey. Last week, I had a physical exam with a new doctor, and she told me not to stress out. FYI, telling me not to stress out stresses me out more. People tried to be super helpful, but unfortunately, they could worsen things. I was not looking forward to being pumped with hormones again, but I endured it a second time. Though it exhausts me, I wanted to give it my best second shot. About a month ago, Micah and I got into it because I went off on how tired I was doing all the work prepping my body while he didn't do a thing to help his sperm get into tip-top shape. I was calm while he was amped up. I intended to convey that I was burnt out on everything. It took a bit of back-and-forth, but Micah finally understood and vowed to do all he could to make this round of IVF successful. Thus, he cut out alcohol, limited his coffee consumption, and worked out more. At least I didn't feel like I was working on this project alone, that Micah also had a significant part to play.

I suppose it is suiting that as I come upon the completion of my memoir about being a new mother, I will begin another fertility journey. It reminds me of a spiral where you come back around but not precisely at the same spot; you hover a level up from where you began with more wisdom.

The Insensitivity of It All

It was a beautiful spring day when a group of us girls went to Geraldine's (a terrific breakfast spot in South Seattle with the most delicious French toast that was basically deep-fried) to celebrate our friend's birthday. We all chit-chatted amongst ourselves, catching up. As we were seated, I was asked whether Micah and I would try for a second. At that moment, I only told three of my closest gfs about my second trial of IVF. Due to my normally not-so-private nature, I decided to divulge. The conversation went something along the lines of this:

Gf #1: Juliet, are you trying for a second or going to try?

Me: Ya, this is all very recent, but I went for a second round of IVF. I had four eggs retrieved, where only one developed into an embryo. The day I was supposed to have the embryo transferred, I received a call as we were parking that it didn't survive.

Gf #1: Oh my god, I am so sorry. I would be so devastated if I couldn't have a second child.

Me: We can still try naturally, but I think we are good right now.

Gf #2 chimes in (has two kids): You seem to have a good balance right now where you can execute your projects. A second may throw things off, and you probably won't have that free time any longer.

Gf #3 decides to add her two cents as well (has three kids au natural): I wanted a girl, so we tried and had another boy instead, but at least we can all say we tried our best. At least we all gave it a shot.

Gf #1 looks at me, embarrassed for gf #3, who was utterly oblivious to her insensitive and unrelatable comments.

Me to gf #3 in the most dignified manner possible: You are lucky to have three healthy, beautiful boys.

We all moved on as if nothing insensitive was ever mentioned and continued our brunching.

Gf #1 texted me after her birthday brunch and felt bad about what gf #3 said—explaining that it wasn't malicious. Blah, blah, blah. Of course, there was no ill intent. The problem was that people thought they could relate or should try to relate to your challenges when they needed to stop right there, and the only response necessary was, "I am sorry you went through that," and that was all. No additional comments needed. Gf #3 could not relate in the slightest and had no clue what fertility assistance was and never will. By the way, her husband was the one who said IVF was unnatural.

I put this up as a post in one of my online mom groups, and many mothers wondered if any of my gfs stood up for me. They did not, but a couple saw my post and felt terrible afterward that they didn't say anything. An insensitive and aloof comment was just that, no matter who was saying it or the intent behind it. It should have been called out. I tried to do it most respectfully and would rather not spend the energy trying to educate gf #3 because it wasn't worth my time. The aloofness and/or self-absorption could be a profoundly innate trait; plus, it was not my job to psychoanalyze her.

39. Lingering Thoughts

Being a new mommy was a planet all on its own. What was imperative was community, a sense of belonging, and true friends who were there to share their experiences and support you in all the ways they could. In a world of insane politics, pandemics, and climate crises, I at least have wonderful girlfriends who I can count on through this parental journey.

At the beginning of my memoir, I posed the question of what a MAM is, but did not provide an answer. At some point, I will be asked to make a blanket statement. Thus, through this writing and research journey, here is my definition:

Modern Asian Mom (MAM): A woman of Asian descent, most likely part of the millennial generation, who formed an embryo (in vivo or in vitro), or adopted, or became a step-mom, and has to navigate through modern-day society, their career, or being a stay-at-home mom (or both). MAMs also deal with Asian family dynamics along with rigid culture and traditions, where their parents unknowingly transferred their trauma into the household, possibly producing a toxic, dysfunctional upbringing. In this modern age, many MAMs have access to more resources, including therapy, support groups, higher education, and an abundance of information available at their fingertips. Thus, MAMs can be more aware of their behaviors and personal issues. Essentially, self-awareness and self-reflection lead to a desire to be more in control of the type of life they lead, so that their children have a better life than they did—one that is more loving, understanding, supportive, and nurturing than one of tough love.

When it comes down to it, many of our parents were immigrants and refugees fleeing a nation they deemed to be unsuitable for the lives they wished to lead. Our parents were in fight-or-flight mode, and survival was the name of the game. They worked hard to build their "American dream" and wanted the same for us. They guided us to the best of their abilities without acknowledging or being able to process their own PTSD and traumas. As we become older and wiser, we realize that we can choose to allow certain energies to enter our bubbles. At a molecular level, DNA comes down to a sequence of sugars and nitrogen bases that carry genetic information. The mutual sharing of these molecules does not permit you to treat them as you wish without consequence. I hope those amid toxic family dynamics can set strict boundaries or cut ties if possible. There were too many posts about this topic on social media where moms felt so guilty. If there is one thing I wish you to remember, it's that you are always your number one priority. Your physical and mental well-being is essential for shaping your child's world and the person they will become. Like my mother always said, "Monkey see, monkey do."

Throughout my fertility journey, I have had two natural pregnancies, two miscarriages, two rounds of IVF, four rounds of IUI, eight eggs retrieved, three embryos, and one live baby. Every single moment, every single penny spent, all worth it.

40. Year 2025 - Dragons, Crabs, and Babies! Oh My!!

<u>Dracarys</u>

As time passes and we age, friendships become more sacred with each new chapter we open. Through my adult years, I have learned what it means to be a good and present friend—a friend who genuinely cares for those who care enough to have a connection with me. Understandably, not all friends will be as close as others, and there are times when friendships become active only due to convenience or the influence of mutual group dynamics. I bring up a particular situation not to publicly point fingers, but because I am still deeply affected by the ordeal, and I hope that all of us can learn from these stories.

Last autumn, I was on an international trip with some close friends. I was placed in a rooming situation (with the opposite sex) that I thought I would be comfortable with, but as a surprise to myself, I was not. It wasn't this person's fault; it was that I am used to sharing intimate quarters with my husband, not other males. After two nights of trying to bear and grin it, I felt the need to communicate my feelings/thoughts to a friend (let's call her Blake), with whom I have known for over a decade, and who I thought would be able to assist me. For context, the friend I was rooming with was brought into the group by Blake. This friend was like the Taylor Swift to her Blake [Lively]. I neutrally and calmly began to discuss my qualms while we were at a store, and perhaps Blake was taken by surprise at first, but what culminated was an experience I will never forget. Instead of actually trying to have an adult, mature conversation, Blake ignored me twice, was somehow distracted by perusing the shelves, and then would walk away. Finally, when I tried to approach a third time, asking if we could discuss my discomfort, I was met with a real-life Khaleesi tyrant (a Game of Thrones reference

182

for those who are unaware). All of a sudden, I was no longer the person with an issue, but I had become the issue. Blake began making accusations, saying I had done this and that, and how I had assumed things. She mentioned that a couple of mutual friends had said negative things about me—she was literally spewing fire from her imaginary dragons. She continued to reign her terror on me until I was depleted, exhausted, apologetic for **her** anger and **her** own assumptions of me. I am not one to easily cry, and I turned into Niagara Falls for most of the trip.

I began piecing the puzzle together, considering our past and present dynamics, as well as things I had heard from our close friends and other parties. A few items were interplaying in the mix. The first thing I came to realize was that Blake had no clue who I actually was, nor would she ever give me the benefit of the doubt due to whatever stories she had heard about me from a couple of her other close friends, with whom I was once close. This was a prime example of her implicit bias, as she never even gave me the chance to tell my side of the story. What was ridiculous was that she blamed me for not coming to her with my version when I had no clue that she had even spoken to any of those friends about these past dynamics. I then began to remember other small, yet telling, encounters with Blake that made it all come into place - I realized that I would never be able to convince her otherwise of the narrative she had molded for me over the years. On this trip, I quickly became the Lannisters.

I tried to understand where Blake was coming from, to empathize, even sympathize with her present life and her potential traumas. In general, I don't think she was content with some aspects of her life. I wanted to understand where all of this anger was coming from, but she wouldn't allow it, saying she wouldn't let me "therapy" her. As close friends, this is exactly what we do for and with each other: act as a form of therapy. This is how we make deeper connections and bonds. Obviously, Blake was not feeling safe enough to explain herself, but I was truly coming from a place of genuine care and love. Instead, I was met with an inferno of gaslighting that I had never experienced before. Basically, I came to a friend for help, and all of it was thrown right back in my face with tenfold the built-up animosity.

Due to the sake of the circle, we ended up "making up" and solved the rooming situation, but the damage was so deep already. I even tried to book an early flight home, but nothing was available. For the next few months, I continued to process the situation and discuss it with a few close friends to gain their insight. Apparently, all was dandy on Blake's end, and she thought we had moved right on. This is another part that added to the dysfunctional friendship dynamics. Just because she felt good about the outcome doesn't mean I felt the same way. I had been traumatized and was trying to console myself. I even tried to give HER the benefit of the doubt on a few occasions, then I came to my own conclusions about the whole debacle and finally decided to put ME first. I continued to harbour these feelings of resentment and realized it was because she never actually apologized for gaslighting me so terribly. I actually don't even think Blake comprehends the extent to which she made me feel or that she dismissed me entirely when I approached her for help. What mattered to her was her reputation and how she could defend her side, so that everyone in our circle would know her perspective. It truly makes me sick to my stomach, actually, that I told her how hurt I was and hoped for acknowledgement of this, to take accountability, yet all she cared about was her own fragile ego and proving she was in the right for her actions.

What was even more astonishing was that Blake began to exclude me from group events and even persuaded another friend that this was okay because it was *her* event she was organizing. Yet, it was a birthday celebration for one of our friends within our circle. Apparently, it didn't matter how much love, energy, time, money, and support I poured into the group for over a decade, because I could be cast aside like I did not matter, as though I was not hurt through her words and mistreatment. I began to really detest her and all of the social media posts I saw of the group without me. What was also painful was that my close girlfriends went along with these events as if everything was fine and dandy. Obviously, I won't ever ask anyone to choose sides, but why did no one call her out on any of this? I believe one or two friends may have, yet the party went on without me, right? It's a touchy situation for all those within the circle, but I do think we are old enough to know what is right and wrong. To be responsible for our behaviours and actions. To set aside egos and pride, especially when a friend tells you that you've hurt them. To speak up even if it causes discomfort. To confront and be mature enough to have an actual conversation when something is bothering you. To move on when you will never receive an apology.

This reminds me of hearing about mothers who gave birth without being able to receive an epidural—they would never do that ever again, but are glad it's over and done with. What I am getting at is that there needs to be something positive gained from an entirely negative experience. I learned that Blake, a longtime friend whom I thought knew me, truly did not. I sat in the dragon den and crawled out with burns. Those who don't know your heart or give you the benefit of the doubt are not your real friends. People who lack actual communication skills don't have the capability to have a mature conversation about certain issues at hand. People project and lash out when they feel threatened or insecure about a part of their life—perhaps when secrets are unknowingly brushed out from under the rug.

Mean girls still exist in adult form because they have not processed their past traumas or continue not to face them. They literally lack the ability to see beyond their reality and perspective. I have surmised that the positives of all this are letting go of a friendship that did not further my growth or make me feel loved/supported. Friends who have not been a genuine cheerleader in your life are the ones who will not stand the test of time. Apparently, some time ago, Blake was speaking to someone I am now fairly close with, who has had negative experiences with her over time. Basically, she noticed either resentment or envy (maybe both?) coming from Blake. They were at an event, and for some reason, I came up, and Blake blurted out that I am not a real doctor. Hearing this made me LOL, and it was just another piece of evidence as to her not being a genuine friend to me ever. She was quietly competing with me apparently and anything I did was taken down in her tiny mental notebook of reasons to hate Juliet. She has also made petty, random comments about other mutual gfs, about their plastic surgery, or how they look terrible in a pic. I was even a victim of these insults two weeks after giving birth to my son. Blake had seen me briefly and then told me I looked like shit. I, of course, let her know that this was completely rude to say to a new mother, and I believe she actually apologized, or at least attempted to.

Recently, I found out that one of my gfs chose me over going to the Lady Gaga concert with Blake and a couple of our friends. Blake exited two of the common group threads, created her own without me, of course, and here she tried to organize yet another event with the circle. These mean girl vibes were off the charts, and another girl actually let her know she was acting in this manner, to which Blake defended herself again, saying that it was *her* event, plus she wouldn't feel comfortable if I was present. It was very telling, the way in which Blake was subtly trying to pull friends to her side—quite childish, really. I felt such gratitude, love, and appreciation for my gf who remembered that I wanted to see Lady Gaga and chose to see the icon with me. Her actions meant the world to me and exude true friendship.

I am at peace with what I accept and don't accept through this transcendence. My main point in all of this is that if anyone confronts you and tells you that you have caused them pain, believe them and apologize. Moral of the story: if you want to put any relationship to the test, go on a week-long international trip. Be sure to bring your dragons.

The Cowardly Crab Pot

For the last decade, I have made it my dedicated mission to uplift, elevate, and highlight my own Asian community and BIPOC in general. I have achieved this through various projects, including casting mainly BIPOC actors for my short film, as well as BIPOC models for published fashion editorials and the runway. I am the founder of Vietology Magazine, where the first edition focused on Vietnamese women and Vietnamese visual artists. Now, I recently published my first book, and within a week of my launch, an Asian woman felt the need to attack my memoir, which is obviously on my fertility journey, navigating being a new mom, and life in general.

To intentionally leave a bad review for an independent, first-time author who is in the red for publishing their own memoir is utterly vile. It is akin to bashing a small Asian-owned business, and instead of being part of the solution, being an actor in the continual problem. I am the sole person in charge of marketing and distribution of my book. It is only available on one platform, and for each physical copy sold, I make a few bucks. My book is in no form flying off any shelves. I am not even making a couple of hundred bucks, mmmkay.

186

What is also astonishing is that this person is from my very own community of modern Asian moms - the crab pot is very alive and well. It's more than disappointing. It is discouraging.

I would have been happy to accept constructive feedback, perhaps through email, where I could also provide context to the issue at hand. However, this person lashed out publicly and anonymously, which I find to be a cowardice act. She tore apart certain portions of my book, thus I don't think she even read the whole thing. It seemed targeted.

Although the review was hostile, I have already incorporated the modifications into this latest version. I thought I was clear originally with my intent, but people love to get on their high horse. Hopefully, the overall reading experience will be improved.

I knew there were risks to publishing and putting myself out there. I am fortunate to have the self-confidence and fearlessness to do so. I spent five years accomplishing this endeavour. Time, money, energy, all while working a full-time career, plus raising a young child and trying to take care of myself, all while also being pregnant again.

Those who wish to make negative comments and tear someone down are truly showcasing the discontent within their own lives. Hopefully, we can all learn from these situations and grow from them. Through the years, I have learned that empathy, consideration, and kindness are essential for living a more peaceful and meaningful life. Maybe we can practice these more and help each other to do so as well.

Hawaiian Delights

It's January, and we are in Waikiki celebrating Tobin and Micah's birthdays. We normally visit the less busy islands, such as Kauai and Kona, but we thought we would switch it up. Tobin had such a blast, and it was nice to be within walking distance of everything. We got our fill of real vitamin D and ate the best poké (btw, Kahala Foodland Market had an incredible selection). It was nice to relax and be carefree for a week. We all had a great time.

Come February, about six days before Saint Valentine's Day, I noticed that I was three days late. I looked at my calendar and it turned out I had ovulated right on Micah's birthday. Let's just say he had received a very intimate birthday gift. In my head, I was like, "No way." Then remembered that Micah normally pulled out but hadn't that night.

When I first envisioned having a family with Micah back when we began dating, I would see a little girl on his shoulders that resembled me. This was why I had assumed Tobin was a girl and was flabbergasted to learn otherwise. Remnants of that little girl energy remained, even as the years passed, even when we thought we were done having kids. Completely happy to be a family of three. In fact, I was already trying to plan a UK Christmas trip. But little did I know, those plans would be shelved for a little longer.

I grabbed a few Dollar Tree pregnancy tests and waited until the next morning to use one, as my sample would be at its highest concentration. The test was positive immediately, and I was astonished. At the age of forty-three, my body churned out a golden egg, ready to be fertilized. Micah's sperm must have been quite jolly with all the fresh Hawaiian goods consumed on our trip.

I showed Micah the test, and he thought I had COVID.

fin.

Photos

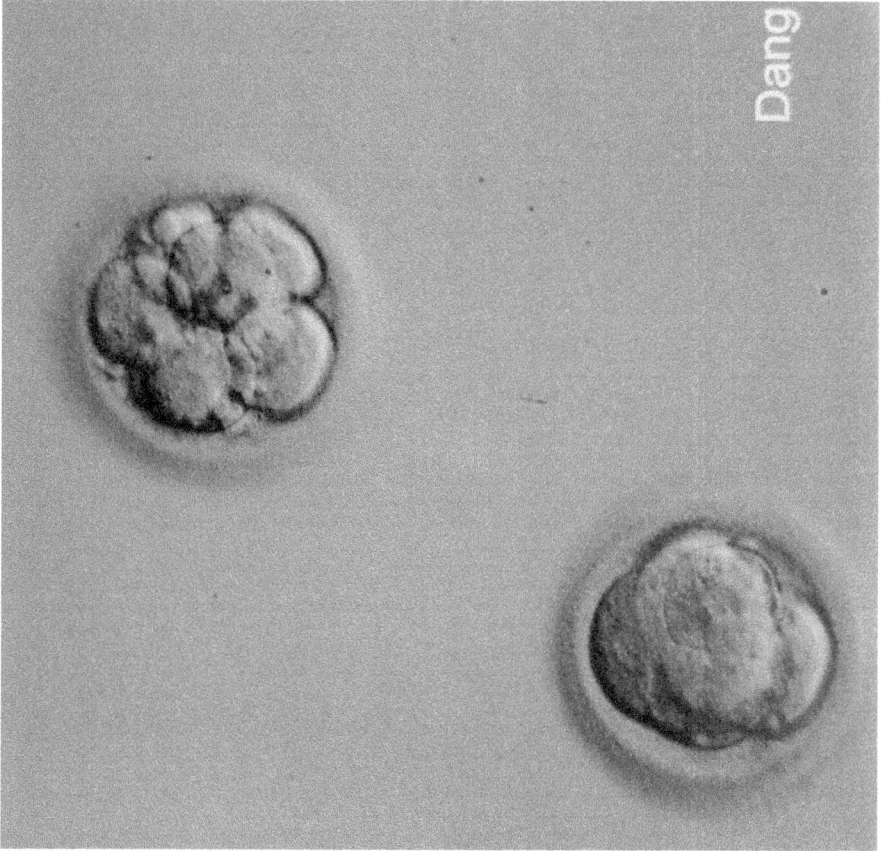

The two viable embryos that were transferred on 4.29.20.

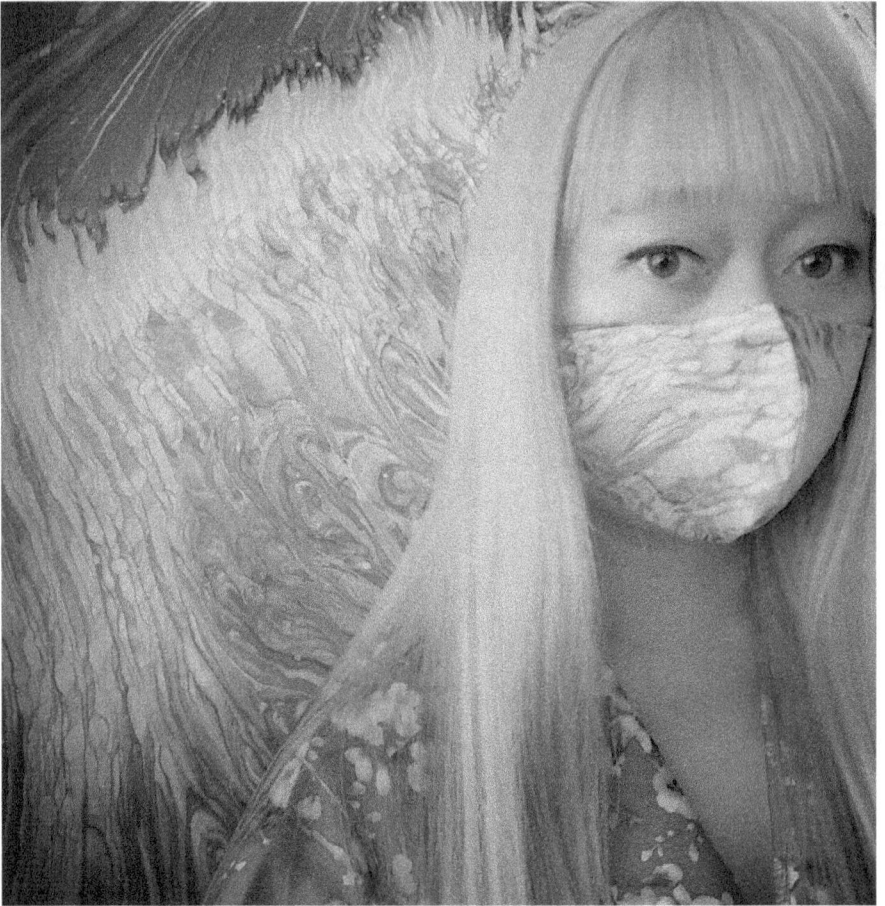
Homemade pandemic masks with my art. July 2020.

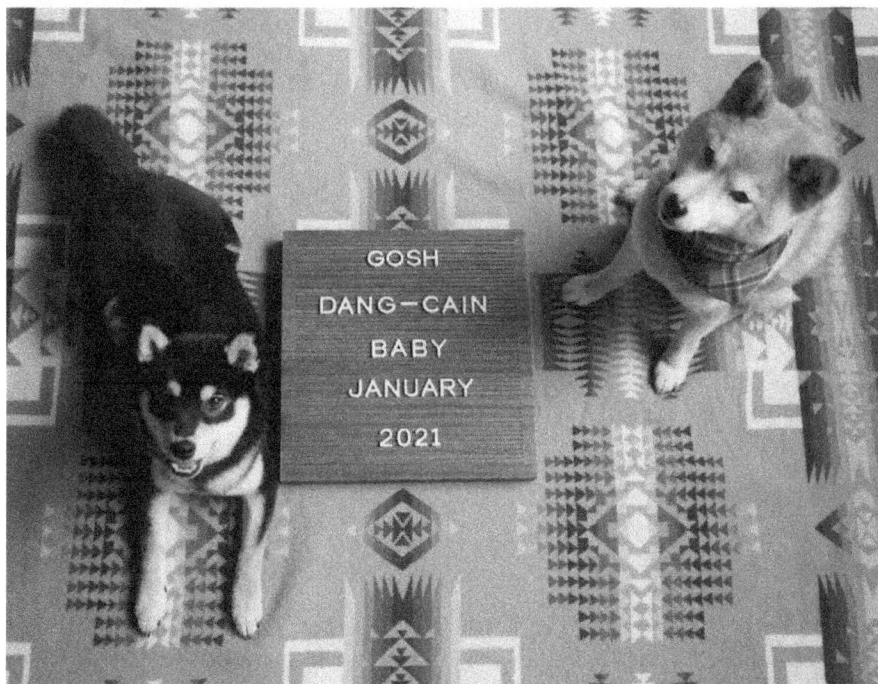

The announcement. August 2020.

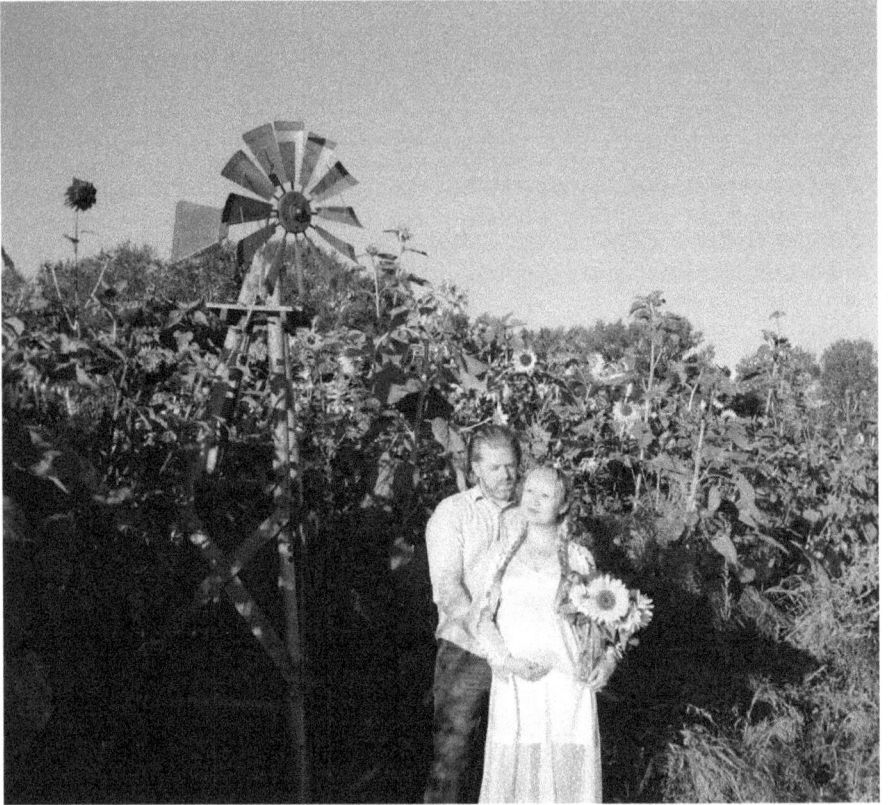

Sunflower fields forever. September 2020.

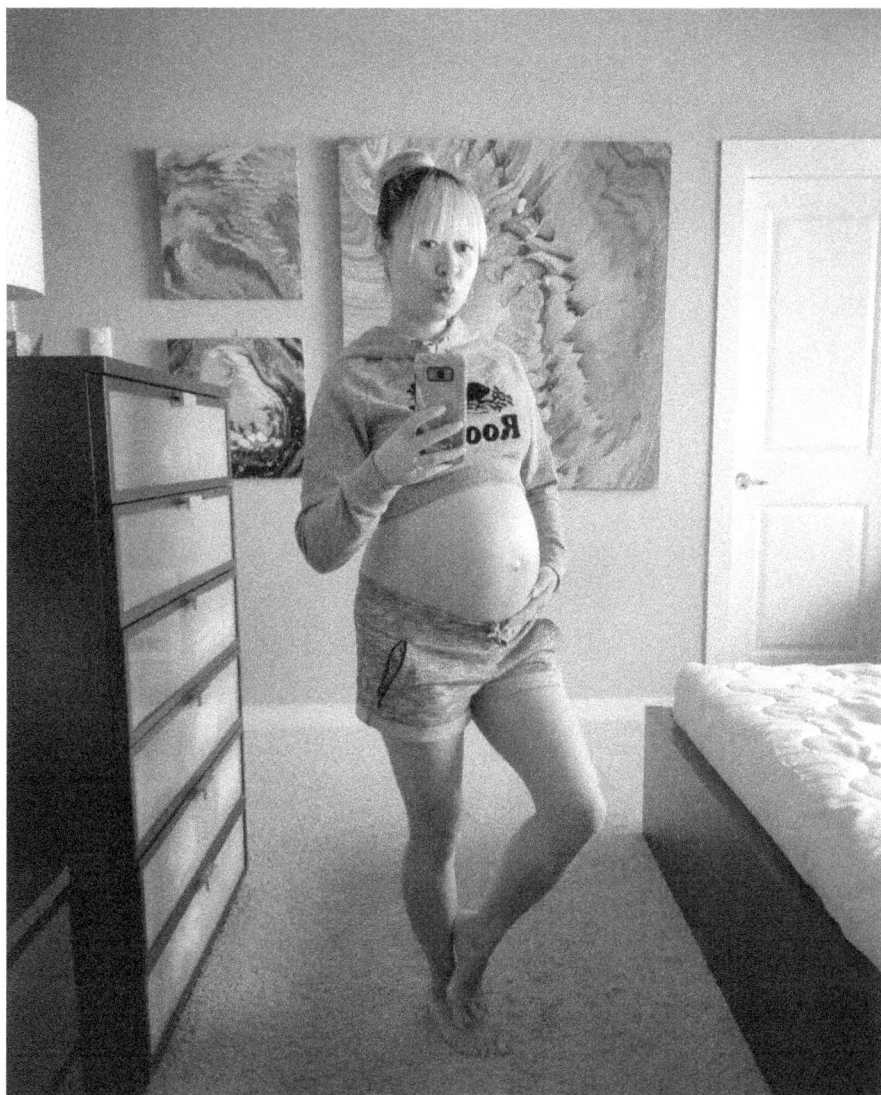

Growing tummy. October 2020.

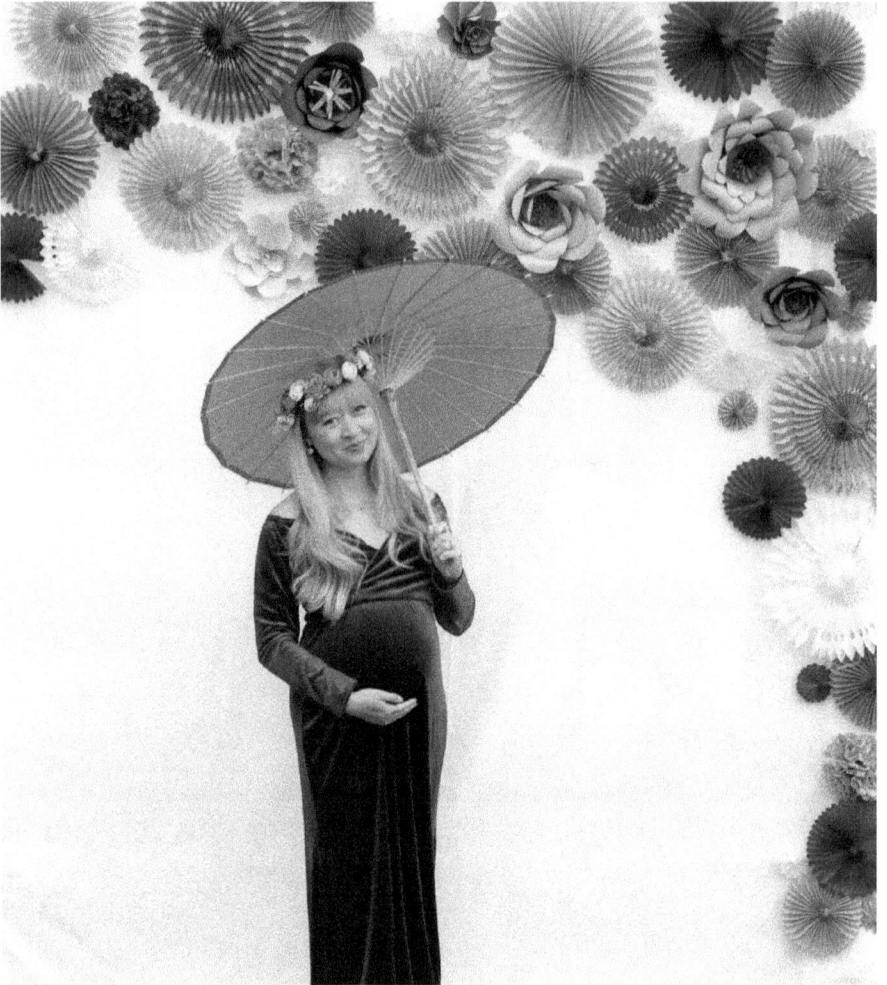

Baby shower bliss. October 2020.

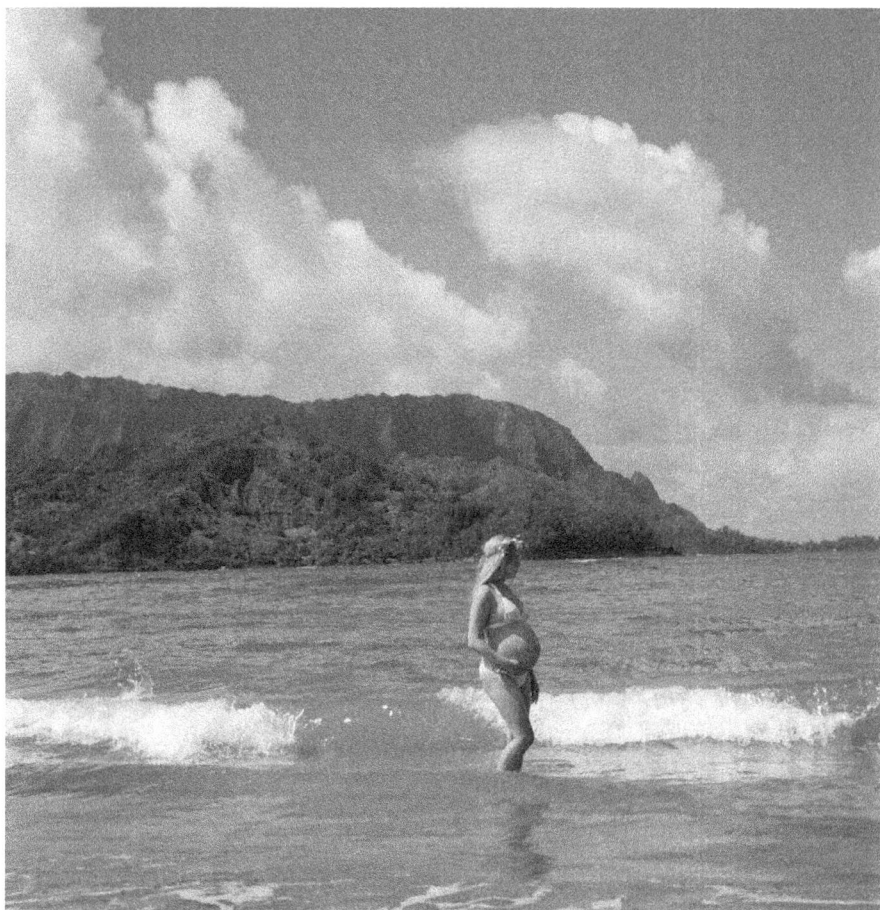
Babymoon in Kauai. November 2020.

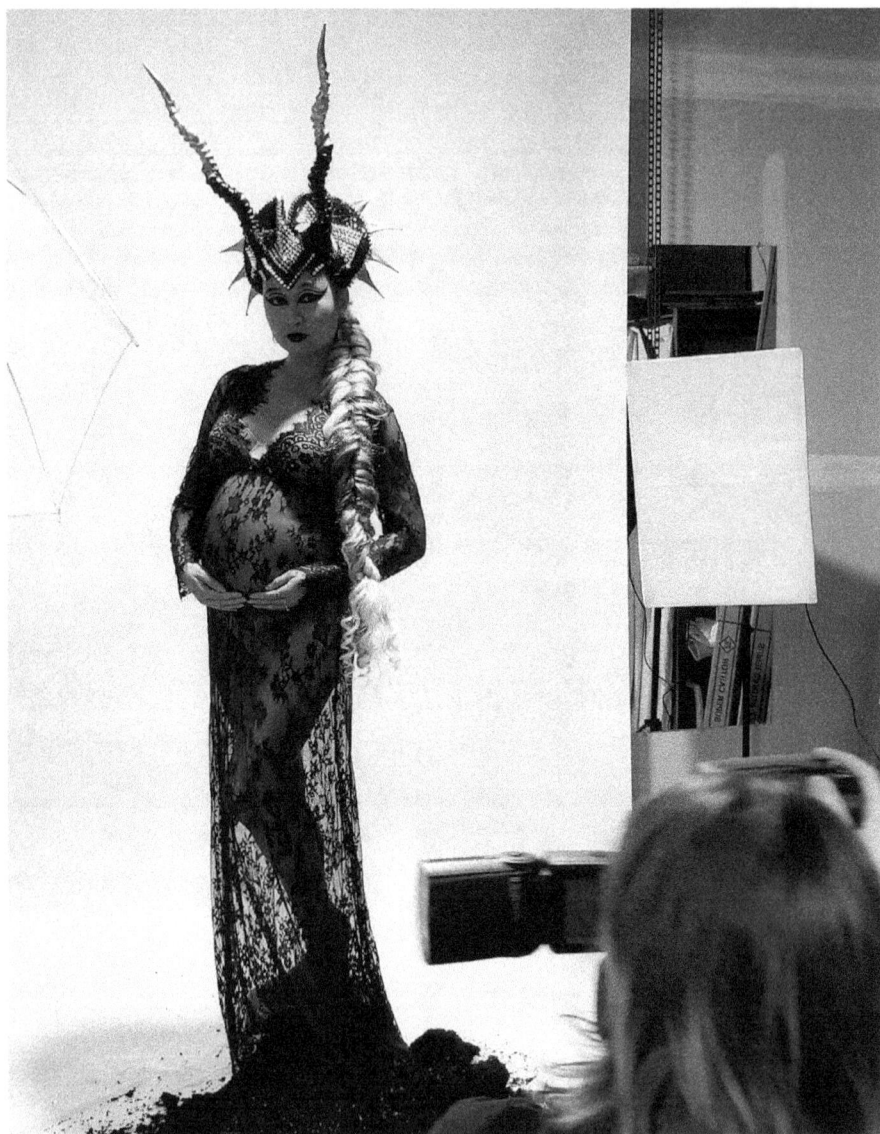
Behind-the-scenes from an editorial pregnant photoshoot. December 2020.

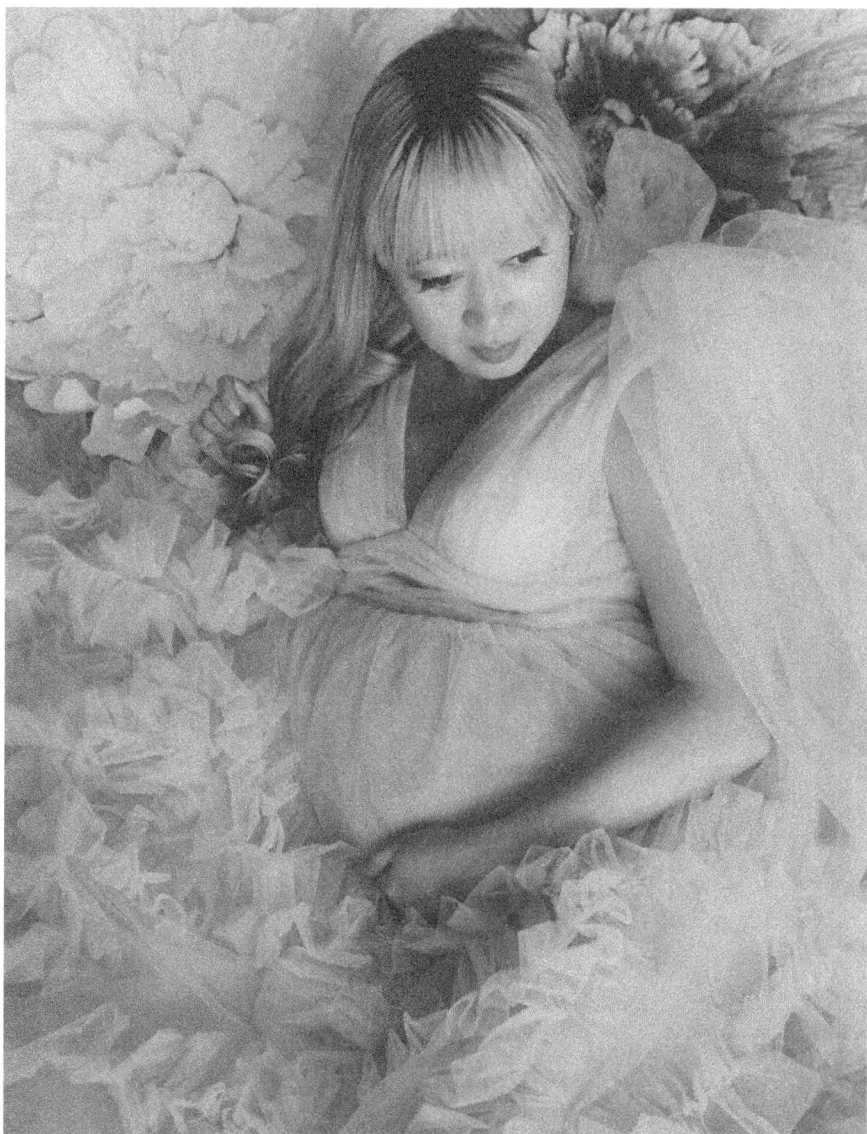
Micah being my IG husband. December 2020.

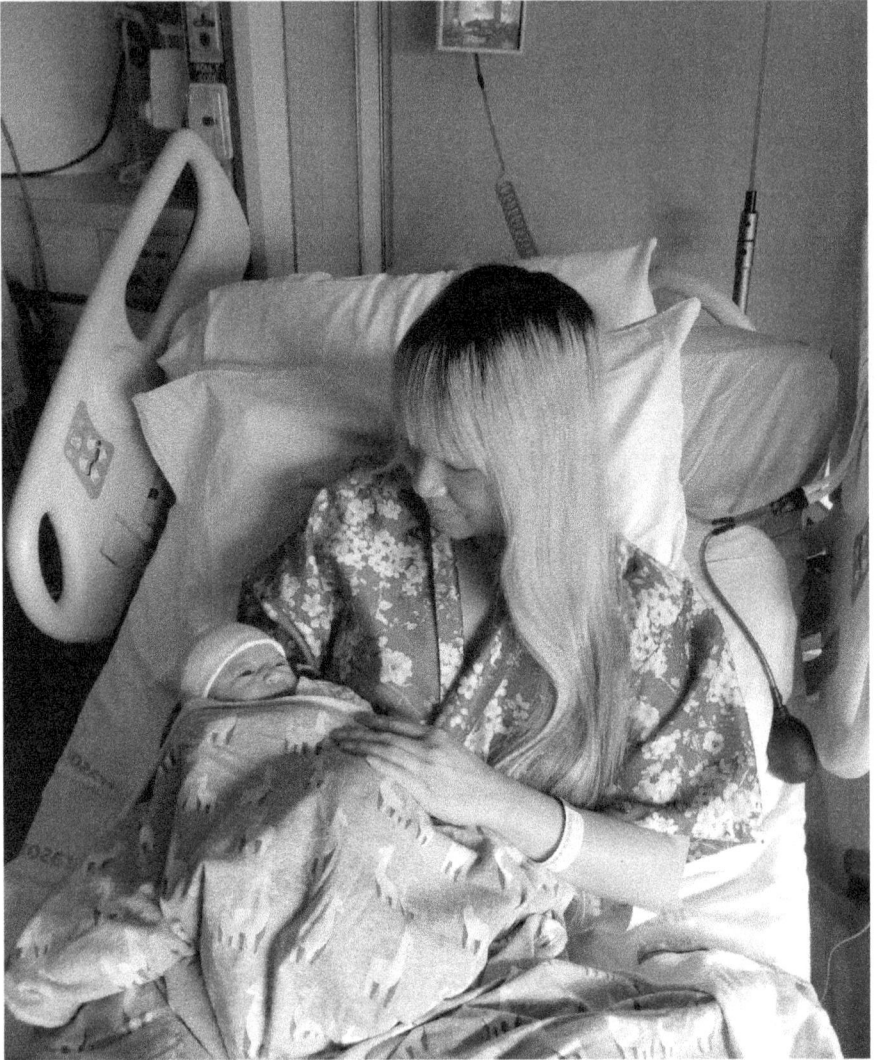
Tobin Dang-Cain is born. January 2021.

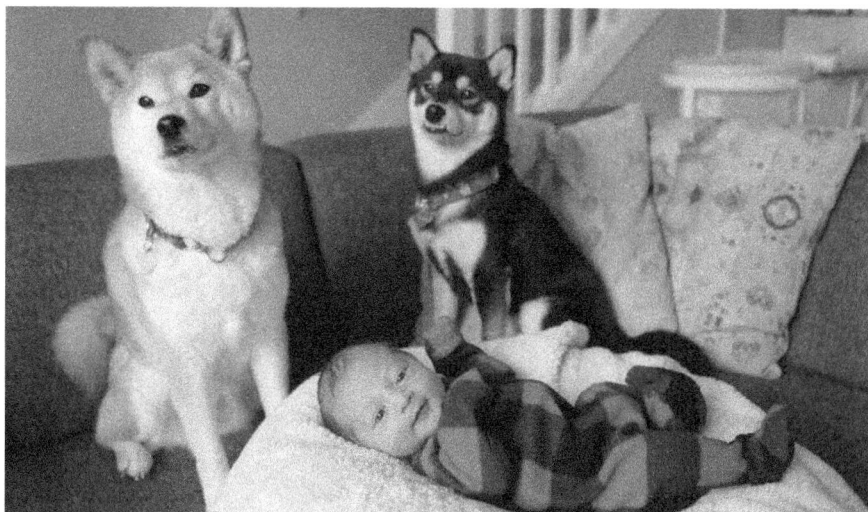
Tobin and the shibes - Yuki & Tomtom. January 2021.

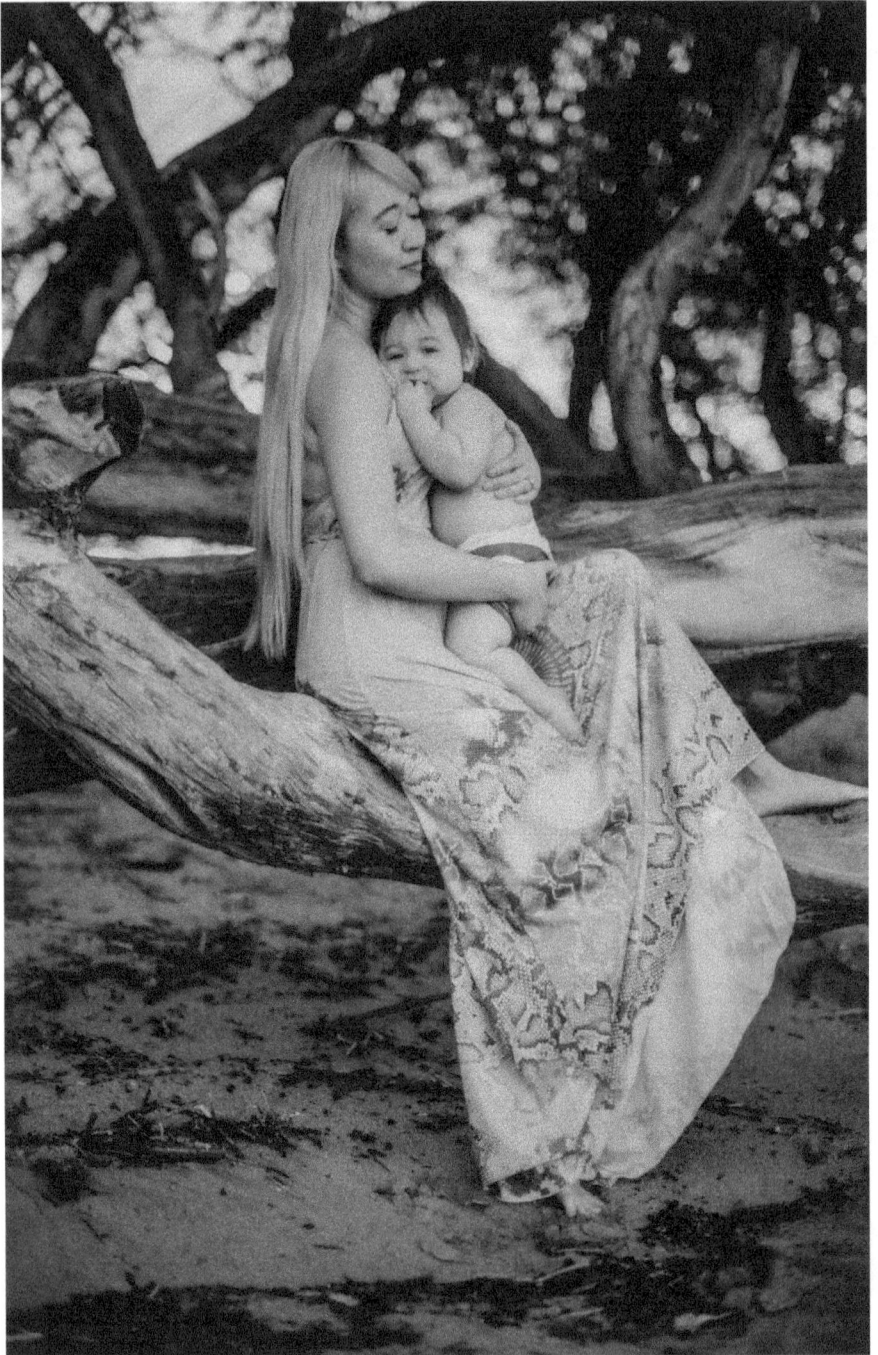

Maui. January 2022.

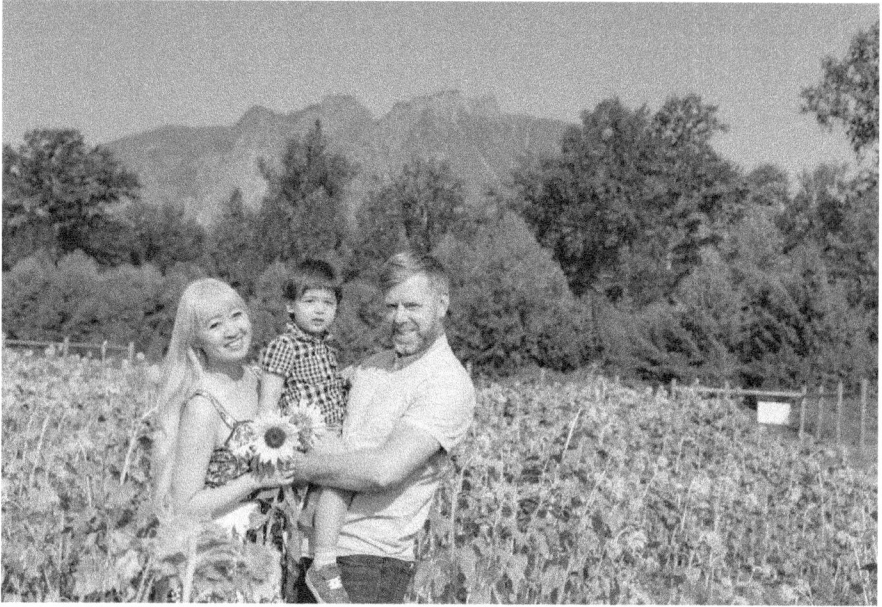

August 2023.

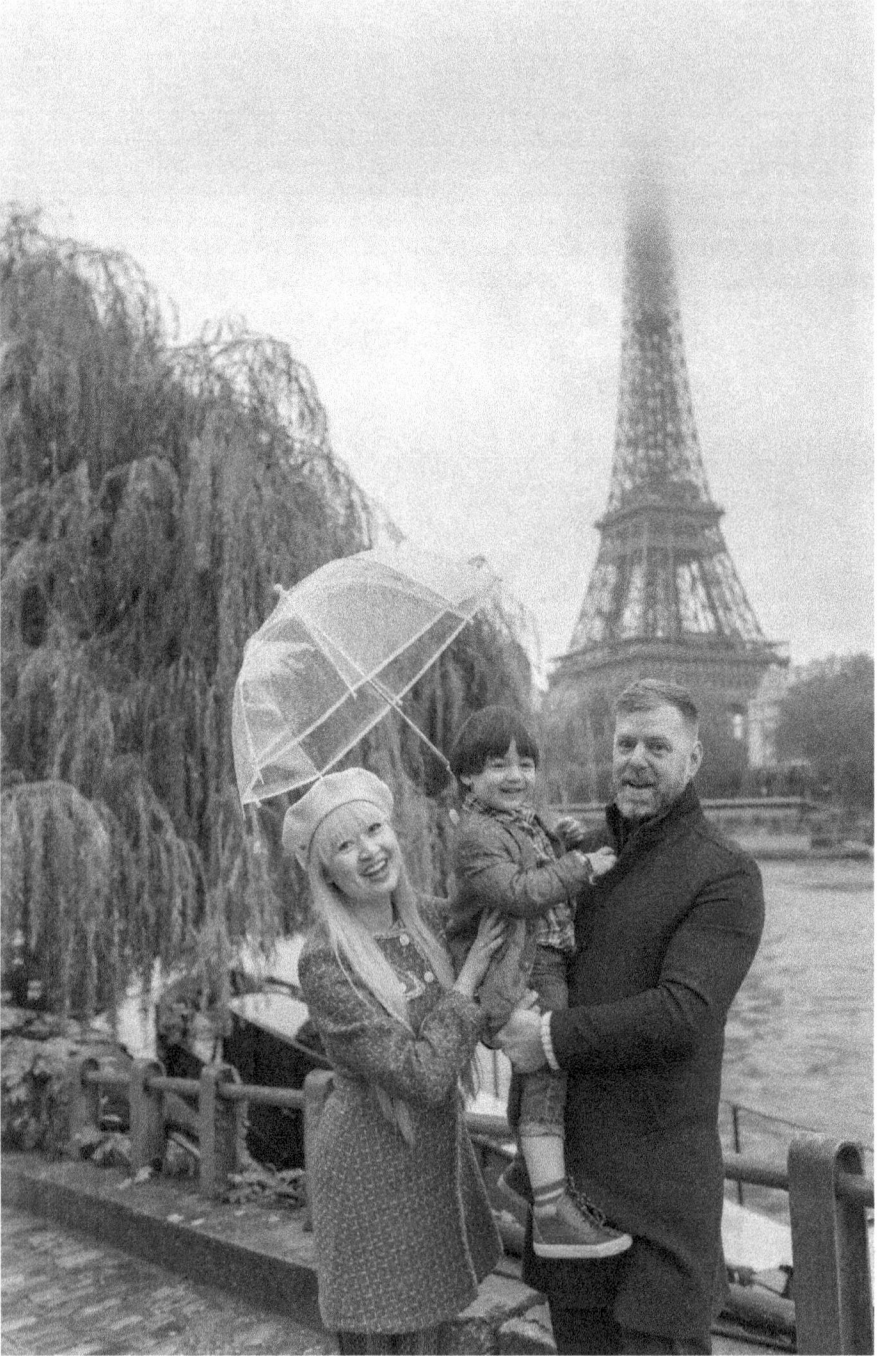

Paris. October 2023.

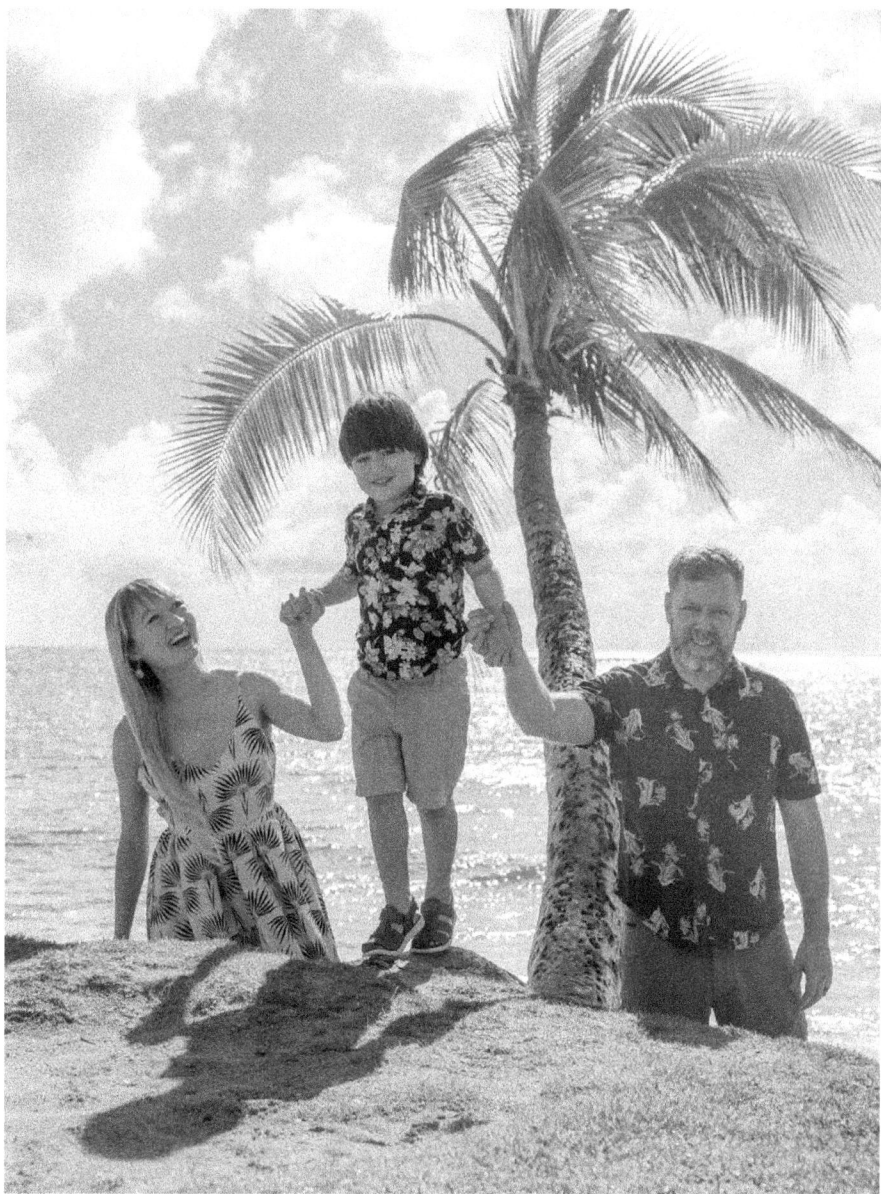

Oahu. January 2025.

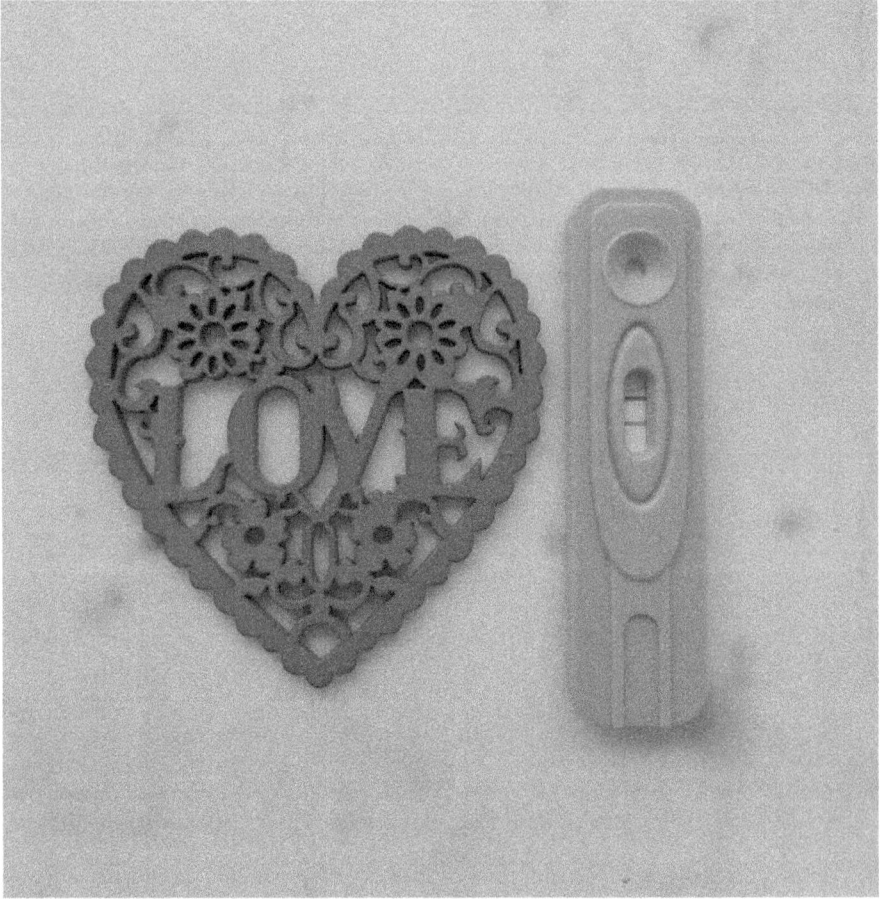

Saint Valentine's surprise gift. 2.14.25

Acknowledgments

I would like to first thank my husband for being the most supportive and loving partner I could ever ask for. I can accomplish my creative projects because he takes care of our toddler and shiba inu.

Thank you to my close friends and family who love me, understand me, and actually know me. Words cannot express how much I appreciate you all so much.

Thank you to my publisher/editor Amy M. Le of Quill Hawk Publishing for guiding me on my publishing journey.

Thank you to my mother who loved me unconditionally and gave me the tools to navigate through life.

MODERN ASIAN MOM

A MEMOIR

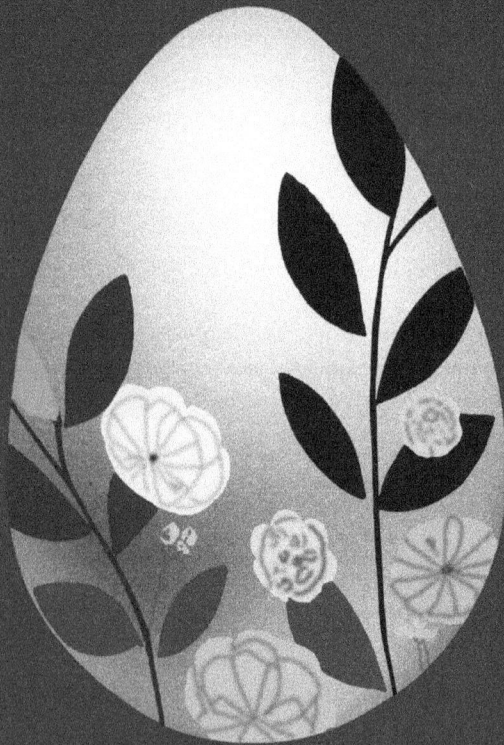

DR. JULIET DANG

About the Author

Juliet Dang, PhD, MS is a Canadian prairie girl who now resides in the Seattle area. She was born and raised in Winnipeg, MB, Canada, where she majored in Biology/Chemistry at U of Winnipeg. After working as a dental hygienist for a couple of years, she moved to Seattle in 2008 to complete a Master's and then a PhD in Oral Biology at the University of Washington. For eight years now, Juliet has been in the medical affairs pharma biotech world and is the subject matter expert on respiratory virus vaccines. In addition to heavily utilizing her left brain as a scientist, Juliet is an artist, actress/model, fashion designer, creative director, editor-in-chief, and producer.

In September of 2024, Juliet made her east coast fashion debut and showcased her ready-to-wear apparel at Asian New York Fashion Week in Manhattan.

Juliet's first major publication was the first edition of Vietology Magazine. The mission and vision was to highlight and elevate inspirational Vietnamese women and Vietnamese visual artists globally. *Modern Asian Mom* is her debut memoir chronicling her fertility journey and life in general.

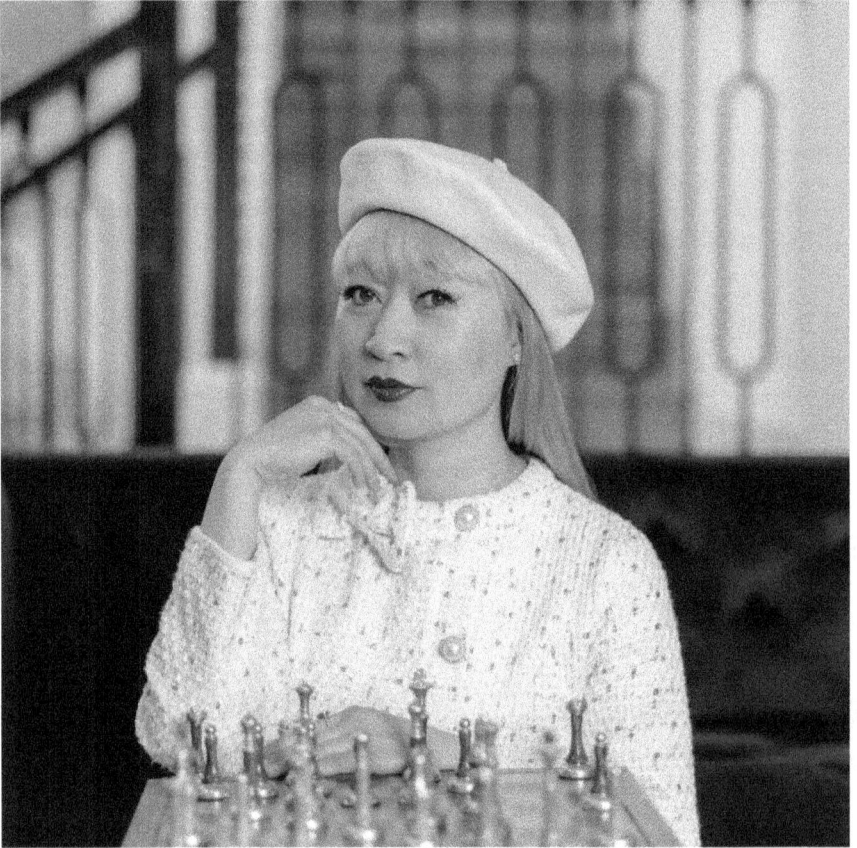
Photo credit - Tero Patana.

www.ingramcontent.com/pod-product-compliance
Lightning Source LLC
Chambersburg PA
CBHW022051020426
42335CB00012B/637